The BrainGate

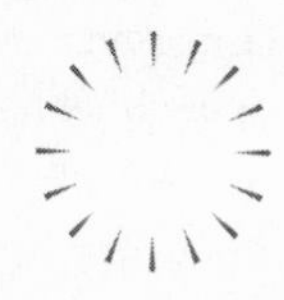

The BrainGate

THE LITTLE-KNOWN DOORWAY THAT LETS NUTRIENTS IN AND KEEPS TOXIC AGENTS OUT

J. ROBERT HATHERILL, PH.D.

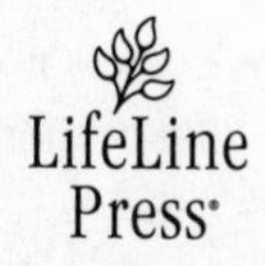

LifeLine Press®

A Regnery Publishing Company
Washington, D.C.

Image credits: pp. 6, 10, 144, 170, Steve Brown; p. 62, Bill Andrews/Custom Medical Stock Photo; p. 160, Art & Custom Medical Stock Photo.

Library of Congress Cataloging-in-Publication Data is available on request.

ISBN 0-89526-141-3

Published in the United States by
LifeLine Press
A Regnery Publishing Company
One Massachusetts Avenue, N.W.
Washington, DC 20001

Visit us at www.lifelinepress.com.

Distributed to the trade by
National Book Network
4720-A Boston Way
Lanham, MD 20706
Printed on acid-free paper

Manufactured in the United States of America

10 9 8 7 6 5 4 3 2 1

Books are available in quantity for promotional or premium use. Write to Director of Special Sales, Regnery Publishing, Inc., One Massachusetts Avenue, N.W., Washington, DC 20001, for information on discounts and terms or call (202) 216-0600.

To Grant Adamson

Contents

Acknowledgments

Many people were vital contributors to *The BrainGate*. I am grateful for the brilliant and scholarly guidance of Dr. Mark Schlenz. I am indebted to artist extraordinaire, Steve Brown. I owe a debt of gratitude to web wizard and scholar Jeff Nelson of vegsource.com. A special thanks goes to Molly Mullen and Mike Ward at LifeLine Press and to Roz Siegal for their inspiration and hours of laboring over the creation of this book. Thanks also to Lauren Lawson and Karen Beck at LifeLine. Finally, I would like to thank the Environmental Studies Program, especially Veronika Banas-Ostendorf, Jo Little, Mary Anderson, J. Marc McGinnes, and Cheryl Hutton for their support of this book.

Part I

Neurotoxicity and Neurotoxic Agents

1

The Brain's Gatekeeper

THROUGHOUT HISTORY, people have been driven by curiosity to explore every aspect of their physical surroundings. Many great frontiers still exist. In space, the farthest galaxies remain a mystery. On earth, the deepest reaches of the ocean await to be studied.

For the human body, the last frontier is the brain. For centuries, this mysterious organ has bewildered many by deftly concealing its multitude of secrets. However, with time, new discoveries and technologies are enhancing our understanding of this complex organ.

The average human brain weighs a mere three pounds and is only the size of a grapefruit. Mostly composed of fat, the brain has no intrinsic moving parts like a beating heart made mostly of protein. Yet it regulates our most basic behaviors—eating, keeping warm, sleeping—and our most sophisticated tasks of music, art, science, and the development of civilization. It cradles our very emotions, hopes, fears, and personality. Despite its immense influence, however, the brain is quite vulnerable, and both inadequate nutrition and pollutants can dramatically affect delicate brain and nervous system functions.

Because of a lengthy and continuing development after birth, human children have the longest period of helplessness in the animal kingdom. Therefore, a baby's brain is a "work in progress." In the first years of life, the brain undergoes profound changes. Shortly after birth, a baby's brain produces many more connections between brain cells than it can possibly utilize. Then the developing organ prunes and eliminates connections seldom used. At around ten years of age, the brain eliminates excess connections and, for better or worse, a set brain pattern emerges. Depriving a child of a stimulating atmosphere can retard brain growth, because the organ itself can wither and suffer permanently. Richly stimulating environments really do produce rich, thriving brains in children and can lessen the risk of brain diseases in adults.

Ironic as it may seem, cell death plays a tremendous role in the pruning process that is vital to brain growth and maintenance. A marvel called programmed cell death, or *apoptosis* (Greek for a flower losing its petals), is vital to a healthy brain. All higher forms of life use apoptosis in normal growth and maintenance. Cells dying because of trauma, invading germs, toxic agents, or lack of oxygen display large invasions of white blood cells from inflammation. When a cell undergoes programmed death in an orderly process, the cell shrivels up and dies quietly, no inflammation occurs, and scavenger cells engulf the debris and recycle it to other living cells.

As it turns out, many drugs and environmental pollutants cause a glitch in cell life by interrupting the tricky process of programmed cell death. Too much or too little apoptosis causes a disturbing pattern of diseases within the central nervous system. The absence of apoptosis increases the risk of cancer and other disorders, since a cell that normally would die lives instead. For example, researchers have linked tumor growth with the loss of a normal, programmed deletion of select cells. Substances that suppress apoptosis will stall the normal neural circuit pruning, and perhaps lead to hyperactive children with excess circuitry. On the other hand, too much apoptosis can destroy vital brain cells that have limited means to form new tissue. Nature uses apoptosis to balance the unbridled growth of cells with the removal of seriously damaged cells.

Development and Stimulation

Clearly, a vital time frame for brain development spans from before birth to about ten years of age. Acquisition of such refinements as motor skills, emotional control, vision, social attachment, language, and logic occurs during certain windows of opportunity. During these developmental windows, a child must be stimulated by proper visual and auditory experiences or risk permanent mental handicap. For instance, researchers have determined that children under the age of ten have an easier time learning a second language than do older individuals. Because the brain circuits have already been hardwired by the time a child reaches ten years, developed brains find it more difficult to learn new languages. But not all windows of opportunity shut at the same time. The developmental window for organizing words in a sentence—syntax—may close as early as five or six years of age, whereas the window for adding new words to a vocabulary may never close.

The hungry brain requires not only proper stimulation, but also things it cannot make on its own, such as oxygen and glucose. Therefore, knowing the brain's essential nutrition is vital to developing the proper diet for optimal adult brain function.

There's much more to eating well than just the pleasure and good company or the flavor of a favorite dish. The type of dietary fat consumed may be crucial to preventing brain disorders. Evidence suggests that the different types of dietary fat may affect a person's mood and ability to learn. Many people are becoming true believers in the old adage "You are what you eat." In terms of brain function what you eat determines both your psyche and intellectual state.

Living with Environmental Chemicals

To encourage optimal function for the adult brain, you must consider both getting critical nutrition and reducing the intake of foods that are detrimental to peak activity of the brain.

After World War II, the production and expanded use of chemicals in the United States created a steady stream of plastics, fertilizers, pesticides, and synthetic fiber products that entered the market. During the 1980s, the National Research Council estimated that a staggering five million different chemical entities had been manufactured by the chemical industry. Today, each year brings to market more than a thousand new or exotic chemicals, adding to an existing stockpile of about 100,000 currently marketed chemicals.

Manufacturing and disposal of these chemicals in the environment have allowed them to enter our food supply and our bodies. Today, we can detect over six hundred different chemicals in people from industrialized countries, most of which were not known or present in humans before the twentieth century. Many experts believe that the presence of even low levels of these chemicals has no significant health effect. Yet widespread use of these chemicals increases even as disorders of the nervous system such as depression, multiple sclerosis, and Parkinson's disease are also on the rise. Further research has linked pesticide use and industrial activities with an increased risk of Parkinson's disease—a particularly devastating brain disorder. People repeatedly exposed to pesticides or who reside near paper mills have an even greater likelihood of developing Parkinson's.

Timeline of Nervous System Diseases from 1800 to 2000

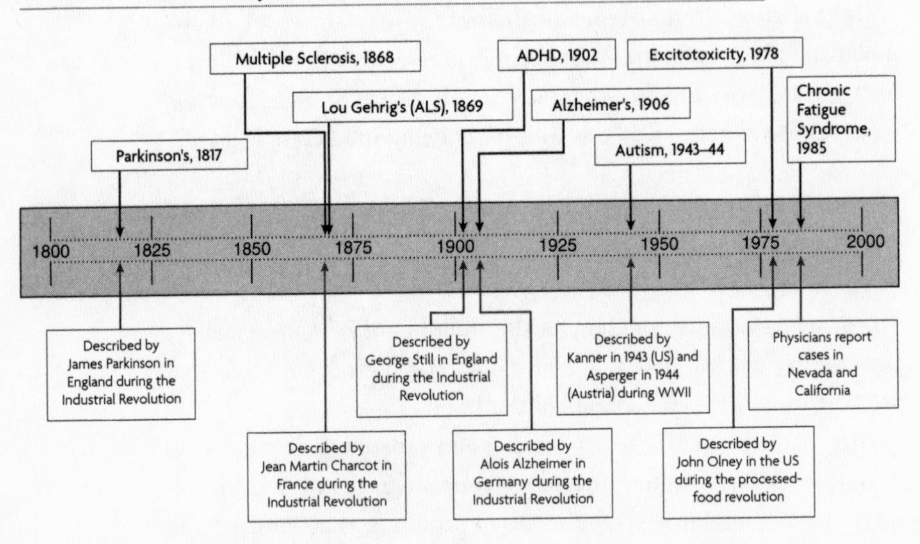

Research published in the *New England Journal of Medicine* showed that pregnant women who transferred higher amounts of chemicals called polychlorinated biphenyls (PCBs) to their infants before birth had more children who developed poor reading skills, lower IQs, memory deficits, and difficulty focusing on tasks. Almost all humans now harbor PCBs in their bodies, a class of toxic chemicals first manufactured by Monsanto in 1929.

Autism, another common learning disorder, surfaced in this country in the late thirties to early forties. Some studies have associated autism with environmental factors, and related learning disorders have shown increased prevalence in children who live near heavily traveled roadways. The incidence of attention-deficit disorder has also increased about 500 percent over the last fifty years.

We might even hypothesize that some people have become vulnerable to Alzheimer's because of slight differences in genetic makeup that allow high-tech pollutants to wreak havoc in the brain.

Silence of the Brain

We know that the brain cannot easily repair itself. Since the brain has limited healing abilities, any damage to most parts of the brain usually results in severe conditions. Intelligent people who ride motorcycles and bicycles wear safety helmets (sometimes aptly named "brain buckets") to guard against brain damage in the case of accidents because they are aware of the risks. But what about less obvious threats to optimal brain function?

Most people don't know that our food, water, and air supply can slowly and silently damage our brains. The depths of the brain do not contain specialized alarm cells to detect pain. Headaches arise from nerve endings in the blood vessels and membranes covering the brain. Brain cells constantly wage microscopic battles for survival, and when they lose, cells die quietly, unnoticed—and you won't even know it until you lose working capacity of the brain. Initial brain cell loss usually doesn't cause problems, because the brain has reserve tissue. If you destroy enough reserve tissue, though, the brain's working capacity becomes severely compromised. For example, Parkinson's disease affects movement and typically shows up in the sixth decade of life. Sometimes, for unknown reasons, Parkinson's disease can strike much earlier, as happened to Michael J. Fox, the charismatic actor who came down with Parkinson's in his late twenties.

Researchers have struggled for more than a century to figure out what causes Parkinson's disease. Until about twenty years ago, our understanding of its causes remained murky; there were few clear clues: no single entity—infection, stress, genetics, or age—seemed to account for the tremors and gradual paralysis of Parkinson's that afflict over 400,000 in the United States alone. Then, in 1982, a series of bizarre events occurred. Since the disease usually occurs in older people in the sixth decade of life, doctors found it strange that young drug users started turning up at hospitals showing signs of Parkinson's disease. Scientists found a toxic contaminant present in the synthetic street heroin being used that caused this strange outbreak of Parkinson's and solved the mystery. "Foreign" chemicals such as pesticides were actually causing Parkinson's disease. An alarming study published in the *Journal of the American Medical Association* claimed that environmental chemicals cause the majority of Parkinson's disease. Other published studies indicated the same troubling connection. While most scientists don't accept it, Parkinson's disease has become the first documented brain ailment of the industrial revolution.

Pollutants that taint our food supply may foster new generations of brain illnesses. Many believe that lead, a highly neurotoxic metal, contributed to the decline of the Roman Empire. In Rome, wine vessels contained lead, and elaborate networks of aqueducts and pipes that supplied drinking water to Rome were lined with lead sheets. Recently, lead has been linked to prevalent learning disorders such as attention-deficit disorder and aggressive behaviors. Several studies have suggested that violent criminals possess elevated levels of lead, cadmium, manganese, mercury, and other toxic chemicals in their systems when compared with nonviolent prisoners.

Many people see growing old as a slow decline into a doddering incapacity. "Going soft in the head" is one of the most unpleasant and frightening features equated with aging. The brain slowly closes down one area at a time, like the floors of a high-rise office building going dark at night. A vision comes to mind of a forgetful and fragile person who struggles to maintain balance by shuffling his feet. Yet with proper diet and lifestyle, this declining course of life need not be the norm in Western society. A growing body of recent evidence shows that through optimal nutrition we can prevent brain disease and boost brain power. Brain wellness requires that we do two important things: lessen our intake of pollutants and receive proper brain nutrition.

The BrainGate

The brain has an important built-in safety mechanism that blocks many items from entering. This blood-brain barrier was first discovered in 1885 in the research of Paul Ehrlich, a bacteriologist and later a Nobel Prize-winner in medicine. His laboratories performed organ-staining studies and observed that blue dyes injected into the bloodstream stained practically every organ in the body except for the brain and spinal cord. Ehrlich's researchers later injected blue dye into cerebrospinal fluid (CSF), the fluid that nourishes and cushions the brain and spinal cord, and found that this time, the dye did indeed stain the brain tissues.

This experiment not only demonstrated the presence of a brain-blood barrier but also showed that no barrier existed between the CSF and brain. Experiments in the 1960s conclusively identified the brain-capillary network as the actual site of the barrier. Scientists soon accepted that a selective brain barrier existed between the blood vessels of the brain. The blood-brain barrier operates on a lock-and-key system; it usually opens only to travelers with the proper keys. Those items that lack a key may approach the blood-brain barrier, but cannot pass through—hence the term *BrainGate*.

The BrainGate forms an encompassing physical barrier and protects the brain from dangerous environments in all vertebrates. The brain needs special protection because it typically cannot recover from damage by regenerating new cells. The normal chemical changes that occur every day in our bloodstream would wreak havoc on the delicate brain without a barrier to protect its delicate internal chemistry. Without a BrainGate, normal activities such as eating and exercising would cause myriad items to enter the brain and disrupt brain cells, allowing them to fire uncontrollably. Seizures and even death would occur. Normal, everyday human life would be impossible without the BrainGate.

Anatomy of the BrainGate

In humans, the BrainGate contains tiny interweaving blood vessels, or capillaries. If placed end to end, the capillaries would stretch for about four hundred miles and cover nearly one hundred square feet of surface area, yet this network occupies less than 5 percent of the brain's total volume.

Anatomy of the BrainGate

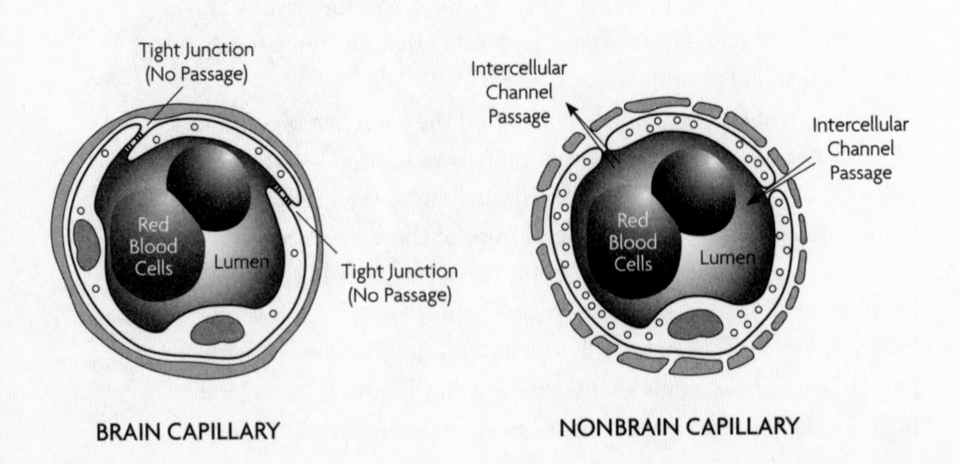

The exclusive BrainGate allows some items to cross, but restricts others from crossing. In contrast to the capillaries in many other organs, brain capillary cells do not have direct channels into the brain, granting the BrainGate a vital purpose. In most parts of the body, cells that line the small blood vessels (endothelial cells) have small channels between each cell so items can move readily between the inside and the outside of the tiny vessels that serve other organs.

It's a different story in the brain. Endothelial cells fit tightly together and restrict items from crossing out of the bloodstream. The BrainGate has tight junctions that seal the margins of the cells that line the blood vessels. Furthermore, while non–brain cells have porous spaces in their basement membranes, brain capillaries have a continuous basement membrane that also restricts compounds from moving out of the blood vessels.

Although most of the brain's capillaries have special features that form the BrainGate, specific localized areas of the brain, such as the circumventricular organs (CVOs), lack a BrainGate. These specialized CVOs control hormones and therefore must be able to measure and respond to their changes in the circulating blood. The hormone messengers must be free to cross into the CVOs, otherwise hormone control will not occur.

O

The BrainGate

Important functions

—Protects the brain from foreign substances in the blood that may injure the brain

—Protects the brain from hormones and brain messengers that would disrupt brain activities

—Maintains a constant internal environment for the brain

General properties

—Large protein molecules do not cross through the BrainGate easily

—Fat-soluble molecules, such as ethanol, environmental pollutants, and barbiturate drugs rapidly cross the BrainGate into the brain

—Molecules that are electrically charged, like proteins, don't usually cross unless assisted by a carrier transporter

A Selective Sieve

The BrainGate is a selective sieve that allows essential substances required for brain activity to cross into the brain. Whether or not a molecule gains entry into the brain depends on several factors, including its size and its ability to dissolve in fat. Because the tiny blood vessels or capillaries have cell membranes made of fats, agents that dissolve in fat pass relatively easily into the brain. Water-soluble molecules such as proteins, hormones, antibiotics, and drugs used for cancer treatment have a much more difficult time crossing the BrainGate. Those items that partially dissolve in both water and fat will slowly seep through the BrainGate, if given enough time. Morphine, for example, behaves this way, and it takes about twenty-five or thirty minutes to cross over. Heroin, a morphine-derived, fat-soluble drug of abuse, crosses the BrainGate about one hundred times faster than morphine.

The fat-soluble hormone estrogen also easily crosses the BrainGate. Estrogen has some very interesting effects on other brain hormones. Many women notice substantial effects of replacement hormone therapy on mood and other physical processes governed by the various control centers of the brain.

The BrainGate permits fat-soluble items to pass easily since it has a large surface area created by its extensive network of blood vessels. However, the brain needs many essential nutrients that don't dissolve in fat, such as glucose and iron. These nutrients enter the brain by the routes of highly selective transport systems. Electrically charged compounds are pulled across the BrainGate by specific proteins that line the inner surfaces of brain capillaries. Some transport systems bring in nutrients like glucose by forming a passage-like opening shaped perfectly to allow the sugar to penetrate the BrainGate. Other transports have selective receptacles or receptors that bristle out into the bloodstream to snare a required nutrient from the bloodstream.

Thus, electrically charged compounds such as proteins cross the BrainGate very slowly, whereas various fat-soluble compounds penetrate so rapidly that some are completely removed from the blood by the brain during a single pass through the brain circulation. The brain absorbs some fat-soluble items so quickly that only the blood flow limits the uptake.

Although fat-soluble compounds can enter the brain quite readily, some electrically charged proteins cannot enter the brain efficiently. For many nutrients, specific shuttles assist in the brain uptake. Because the brain uses glucose almost exclusively as a fuel, glucose shuttles richly endow the BrainGate.

Another prominent transport system in the BrainGate enhances the uptake of large neutral amino acids used to make proteins and brain messengers that transmit signals in the brain cells. This amino acid shuttle has the capacity for transporting at least ten different amino acids present in the blood. These multiple amino acids will thus compete with one another for transport into the brain. Consequently, when one amino acid rises in the blood, it can reduce the uptake of other amino acids. Such imbalances may play a role in the brain damage found in conditions such as phenylketonuria and excitotoxicity.

The human brain evolved with a diet that provided a steady release of amino acids from digestion. The brain uses amino acids to make neurotransmitters, or brain messengers, agents that transmit signals. But modern food-processing techniques have drastically altered the limited availability of amino acids by adulterating food with free amino acids in the form of monosodium glutamate (MSG) and by adding digested (hydrolyzed) animal and plant proteins. Processed-food manufacturers use these procedures to increase flavor, change food textures, or increase the food's shelf life.

O

The BrainGate can be weakened and compromised by

—Mental stress
—Bacteria and viral infections
—Ionizing radiation (such as in medical or dental X-rays)
—Microwave radiation (such as in cell phones, antennas, microwave ovens)
—High blood pressure (more damaging substances cross the blood-brain barrier in people with high blood pressure)
—Developmental stage (the BrainGate is not fully formed at birth and not fully developed until adulthood)
—High concentrations of a given substance (for example, the sugar mannitol given or consumed in excess)
—Mechanical trauma
—Lack of oxygen
—Inflammation

The problem with eating "free" amino acids or those that don't need digestion is their rapid uptake in the brain. A recent dietary cause for brain cell death involves excessive stimulation, or excitotoxicity, of the brain cells by one particular amino acid—glutamate. Many different foods contain glutamate. Every cell in the body makes glutamate. The brain transports and stores glutamate for use as a brain messenger—a chemical signal that allows one brain cell to talk to or have a dialogue with another. Such brain cell conversations underlie the basic operations of the brain. Glutamate is the most common amino acid used to make brain messengers. Glutamate does have an ugly side, however: excessive amounts of glutamate will rapidly kill cells in the brain and spinal cord. Normally, nerve cells prevent the buildup of glutamate by using glutamate transporters that vacuum up the excess glutamate around cells. Excess glutamate constantly stimulates the nerve cell and can even overstimulate it to the point that the nerve cell dies.

The workings of the BrainGate are far more complex than just a barrier wall. It has specific shuttles that help in the uptake of important nutrients and hormones and actively pumps items out to control the buildup of toxic substances within in the brain. Enzymes present in the BrainGate alter or disarm brain messengers, drugs, and toxic agents before they can enter the brain and disrupt function. As a result of these diverse functions, the BrainGate can effectively supply the brain with the nutrition it requires and protect it from toxic agents while maintaining a proper nutrient balance.

Besides taking steps to ensure your overall physical health, you can now add essential nutrients and adopt lifestyle factors that not only support brain health, but also preserve brain function. As the general population ages, the number of people afflicted with brain diseases will rise. This book will help you lower your risk of brain illnesses.

2

Traffic Control

Letting in the Brain Boosters

WHETHER THE BRAINGATE permits an item to pass depends upon the item's size, electrical charge, and ability to dissolve in fat. Because the tiny blood vessels or capillaries have cell membranes made of fats, things that dissolve in fat pass more easily into the brain. Water-soluble substances such as many antibiotics, cancer drugs, proteins, and many hormones have more difficulty gaining entry.

Gaining Entry Through the BrainGate

Because the brain also needs essential nutrients—such as glucose and iron—that don't dissolve easily in fat, the BrainGate pulls them through with special shuttles that line the inner surfaces of brain capillaries. Some shuttles bring in nutrients like glucose by forming a passageway perfectly shaped to allow glucose to pass. Other shuttles have selective receptors that act like padlocks that extend out into the bloodstream and require a key before allowing an item to cross the BrainGate.

The Brain's Shuttle Delivery System

The BrainGate shuttles are similar to a turnstile used by people to enter a ballpark. Before the ball game, the turnstile can become clogged with too many people entering the stadium all at once. The BrainGate can also become clogged with items that share the same turnstile (or shuttle). Dietary items present in excess swarm the turnstile and block others from crossing the BrainGate. What you eat is directly responsible for what gets in line at the BrainGate. Because the brain requires glucose as its primary fuel, the BrainGate is richly populated with glucose shuttles. The cells that make up the BrainGate contain large levels of cholesterol compared with other areas of the body. Cholesterol gives the BrainGate a rigid form, making transport across it more difficult.

The BrainGate maintains the proper environment for the brain to work and shields the brain from toxic agents. Items in the blood that cross rapidly into the brain include glucose (a vital source of energy), ions like sodium and potassium (used for electrical activity), and oxygen (for producing energy). Small molecules, like ethanol, also easily cross through the BrainGate. We know that some water-soluble molecules such as amino acids, choline, purine bases, nucleosides, glucose, and L-dopa (used to make dopamine) pass into the brain carried by special shuttles located in the BrainGate.

Items turned away from the BrainGate include large proteins and many antibiotics. Oxygen and carbon dioxide readily cross the BrainGate, as do alcohol, caffeine, amphetamines, cocaine, heroin, and nicotine. Hormones like estrogen also gain easy access to the brain and are able to act on brain messengers to produce stimulating effects in the brain.

The brain protects its fat from turning rancid (a process known as lipid peroxidation) by drawing antioxidants such as vitamins C and E, carotenoids, lycopene, and bioflavonoids across the BrainGate. Some antioxidant plant pigments, such as the proanthocyanidins from dark-red or blue fruits like blackberries and blueberries, can help slow the progress of some brain diseases. But the BrainGate will also exclude some potentially beneficial items. So because the BrainGate is so selective, proper nutrition is critical to brain wellness.

Substances with electrical charges such as glucose and amino acids must depend on special shuttles to cross into the brain. Because the brain primarily uses glucose for energy, the BrainGate contains areas richly populated with glucose shuttles. The brain needs a steady restocking of glucose, and if the blood glucose levels drop quickly, so will the brain glucose levels. A sufficient and steady level of glucose circulating in the blood is the only way to keep the brain supplied with glucose.

Large Neutral Amino Acids (Phenylalanine, Glycine)

The BrainGate shuttles raw materials for making brain messengers and proteins such as large neutral amino acids (LNAA). In stark contrast to the glucose shuttles, which only transport glucose and vitamin C, the LNAA shuttle can transport at least ten different amino acids that circulate in the blood. Because ten different amino acids use the same shuttle, they compete for entry into the brain.

For example, LNAAs compete for one common shuttle, and some LNAAs (like phenylalanine) have a stronger attraction to the shuttle, so they occupy more than 50 percent of the shuttle seats. Simply increasing one specific LNAA above normal dietary levels may elevate the brain levels of that particular amino acid.

This strong attraction, or "high affinity," for the shuttle vehicle varies from one LNAA to another. From the strongest to the weakest these LNAAs include tryptophan, phenylalanine, leucine, tyrosine, isoleucine, and methionine. Unlike other amino acids, tryptophan attaches to a protein in the blood, making it too large to cross the BrainGate. Tryptophan has to fill up the proteins before unattached tryptophan can be presented at the BrainGate. Because of this mechanism, tryptophan must be eaten in high amounts to dramatically increase the brain levels.

Competing amino acids need to be balanced. Recall that diet alone dictates how much of the assorted amino acids are presented to the BrainGate. Too many excitatory amino acids will storm the BrainGate and more will cross into the brain, increasing the chance of excitotoxic damage.

When you eat a diet rich in one specific amino acid, that amino acid swarms the turnstile and more of it will cross the BrainGate. The assorted amino acids turn into different brain messengers once they enter the brain. Diet, therefore, plays a critical role in the balance of different brain messengers. In turn, various brain messengers play huge roles in moderating mood and brain activities (see Unlocking the BrainGate on page 108).

We now know for sure that the BrainGate has many shuttles in addition to those for glucose and amino acids. Special shuttles transport other important substances, including thiamine, pantothenic acid, biotin, vitamin B6, riboflavin, niacinamide, carnitine, inositol, sodium, potassium, some hormones and other peptides, purines, and nucleosides for nucleic acid synthesis.

Enemies at the Gate

Because the BrainGate controls the movement of so many substances into the brain, some vital nutrients may have difficulty getting through the BrainGate and need help to gain access to the brain. We know that many nutritional items gain access to the brain by specialized shuttles. Some toxic agents, however, exploit this mechanism and actually piggyback onto different shuttles to gain entry to the brain.

Mercury

The neurotoxic metal mercury can fool the BrainGate. Methylmercury can combine with the amino acid cysteine, which forms a structure similar to the amino acid methionine, and is then transported into the brain by the LNAA-system shuttle. Dietary fiber can assist in the removal of mercury, since bile is the major route of elimination.

Aluminum

Another weakness of the BrainGate concerns aluminum transport into the brain. Aluminum will gradually build up in the bones and brain tissues. Aluminum can cross the BrainGate like a "Trojan horse." Because aluminum and iron share some common chemical properties, aluminum crosses the BrainGate by impersonating iron and using the iron shuttle. Greater brain uptake of aluminum might also be made possible by an increased leakage of the BrainGate as a result of diseases such as high blood pressure (hypertension) or Alzheimer's.

Iron

In excess, iron can help form toxic free radicals that turn fats rancid. We also know that high levels of iron are often found in the brains of people afflicted with diseases such as Alzheimer's and senile dementia.

Aspartame

Eating foods with added aspartame can lead to increased blood and brain levels of phenylalanine. High brain levels of phenylalanine are known to disrupt the enzyme tyrosine hydroxylase, which is responsible for making the mood enhancers serotonin, dopamine, and norepinephrine. A diet rich in aspartame-sweetened foods may have two harmful effects: By increasing the phenylalanine in the blood, tryptophan will have to compete and less will enter into the brain. Less serotonin results from lower levels of tryptophan in the brain. Serotonin calms the nerves. In addition, high levels of phenylalanine in the brain will result in less production of other key brain messengers like dopamine and norepinephrine, both of which are critical to mental activities.

Prescription and Nonprescription Drugs

Blood proteins can ferry a lot of toxic chemicals around the body, which actually benefits you because the proteins keep some of the toxic chemicals tied up and unable to break free and cause harm. Pollutants attached to proteins become too large to cross the BrainGate.

Many common drugs also grab on to these same blood proteins and kick the toxic chemicals off, thereby freeing them to cause harm. Only the unbound, free form of the pollutant is capable of crossing the BrainGate. Therefore, limit your use of common over-the-counter and prescription drugs, since they burden the clearance system for removing pollutants from the body and may very well increase the blood levels of free toxic agents presented to the BrainGate.

Weaknesses of the BrainGate

Circumventricular Organs

Small, distinct areas of the brain called circumventricular organs (CVOs) monitor various body functions by detecting the blood levels of hormones and other signaling chemicals that don't cross the BrainGate. One CVO, the hypothalamus, controls food intake and must monitor the blood levels of hormones such as insulin, which cannot cross the BrainGate. Because of their unique functions, the CVOs need to allow passage of many compounds and are located outside the protective fenced areas of the BrainGate.

Neurotoxic agents that normally can't get into the brain freely cross into the CVOs. The food additive monosodium glutamate (MSG) is particularly toxic to the CVOs. MSG causes toxicity to brain cells by literally exciting them to death. MSG produces many toxic effects on the CVOs and alters such things as brain messenger levels, metabolism, and insulin levels in the blood.

Animal studies have discovered an alarming trend. Animals given MSG became extremely obese, even though they were not eating additional food. The underlying reason MSG caused obesity seems related to a loss of controlling insulin levels. The MSG-treated animals showed persistent high levels of blood insulin, which stimulates the body to make and store fat rather than build lean body mass.

The implications of the MSG studies are alarming. Apparently, a constant diet of processed foods containing MSG can damage critical areas of the brain that regulate food intake and fat production.

Cargo Delivery in the Nerve Cell

In some brain diseases or in cases of trauma, spots or patches made of cast-off debris called plaques deposit in brain tissue. These brain plaques are often made from a protein called amyloid-beta. We know that plaques form even in the brains of healthy people as they age. They can also appear after head injuries from boxing. But why do amyloid-beta plaques overrun the brain in Alzheimer's disease? All cells in the human body make amyloid-beta but only brain cells seem to be harmed by its presence.

To answer this question we need to look at nutrient delivery in the nerve cells and other players that form plaques and deposits leading to Alzheimer's. Another protein called amyloid precursor protein (APP) gets chemically chopped up and frees amyloid-beta. APP is a protein involved in transporting materials within the nerve cell.

The nerve cell cargo delivery (called axon transport) operates like the air-pressure system that banks use at their drive-up windows to shuttle transaction documents through tubes to and from your car. Air pushes and pulls the plastic document container down the tubes in a way similar to how the cargo transport protein (APP) works. Now, APP works fine until it meets the wrong sushi chef, who chops APP incorrectly. Then amyloid-beta fragments fall off like so much plastic roadside litter. If enough amyloid-beta fragments build up and clog the roadway, the resulting debris or plaques stall the cargo delivery.

Toxic metals like mercury can also ruin the road surface and stall the cargo transport. If the cargo isn't delivered, the cells are deprived of critical proteins, signals, and fuel. We know that cells with a low fuel supply trigger cells to commit suicide. This is especially harmful to brain cells that have limited abilities to replenish themselves. Just like a busy freeway, a number of glitches can result in clogged roads and stalled cargo delivery within the nerve cells.

Flavonoids: Antioxidant Protection for the BrainGate

Flavonoids are a class of plant pigments that consist of over four thousand natural compounds found in most fruits and vegetables. Flavonoids are not considered essential nutrients, yet many keep inflammation in check and strengthen blood vessels and connective tissues.

Some of the different categories include:

- Anthocyanins, the red-blue pigments, are found in red and dark-blue fruits, like grapes, raspberries, cherries, blueberries, blackberries, and plums.
- Flavonols, which include catechin compounds, are found in green tea, and the proanthocyanadins and Pycnogenols, which are found in pine bark and grape seeds.
- Flavones, which include quercetin, are found in onions and garlic. More than one hundred and thirty-five different variations of quercetin have been isolated. A very common variety is rutin, used to treat blood capillary fragility. Citrus fruits are also a rich source of flavones and flavanones.
- Isoflavonoids, which are found in legumes such as soybeans and soy products.

Flavonoids Stabilize Collagen in the BrainGate

Flavonoids block the breakdown of collagen and prevent oxidation. Collagen is the most common connective tissue in the body. At least five types of collagen make up connective tissue in many parts of the body: the bones, skin, teeth, tendons, ligaments, fascia, cartilage, and connective tissue in organs such as the liver and kidneys. The outermost layer that surrounds the capillaries (basement membrane) in the BrainGate is made from strong connective tissues such as collagen; fibronectin, a protein that attaches to and strengthens collagen; and laminin, which acts like mortar in a brick wall.

A step-by-step process makes collagen, and every step requires vitamin C, a critical vitamin for brain health. In fact, the brain concentrates vitamin C levels to 10 to 100 times that of the levels found in blood. Collagen uses flavonoids to prevent free radical damage and inflammation.

A number of flavonoids such as catechin from green tea have been shown to stabilize collagen. In addition, catechin stimulates the manufacture of collagen and makes it less prone to breakdown by blocking the enzyme that degrades collagen.

Other flavonoids, such as anthocyanins and proanthocyanidins, also foster collagen formation and stability. Anthocyanins contained in the European blueberry, or bilberry, preserve collagen by increasing collagen formation and cross-linking. Collagen will attach to nearby collagen molecules, or cross-link, which strengthens collagen much like right-angle supports do in a wood-framed house.

A number of animal studies show that flavonoids in blueberries and grape seeds can strengthen the BrainGate when exposed to agents that are known to weaken it.

A series of animal studies used collagenase and dimethylsulfoxide (DMSO) to damage the collagen in the BrainGate. Animals first treated with flavonoids (anthocyanoside) showed less BrainGate damage and leakage after getting DMSO. Flavonoids virtually eliminated the increased brain leakage that occurred with DMSO. In addition, the flavonoid groups completely recovered BrainGate activity in twenty-four hours after being exposed to the collagen-weakening agent. On the other hand, animals not receiving flavonoids required seventy-two hours for the BrainGate to return completely to normal. Flavonoids protected the barrier-like structure even when faced with compounds known to harm the BrainGate.

Other experiments created greater seepage across the BrainGate by using high blood pressure (hypertension), which is known to cause leakage across the BrainGate. As you get older this becomes especially true. Think of a garden hose: the greater the water pressure, the more likely the hose will leak. Older garden hoses spring leaks easier since parts of the hose are worn and degraded. Once again, animals first treated with flavonoids showed normal leakage typically seen in the absence of high blood pressure or with normal blood pressure.

Flavonoids Reduce Inflammation

Inflammation also causes the BrainGate to leak. In addition to protecting the BrainGate membranes, flavonoids have another protective feature: they reduce inflammation. Anthocyanosides in particular lessen inflammation and block free radical toxicity. These actions can be significant in reducing capillary leak and further inflammation. Thus flavonoids are an extremely vital dietary component that strengthens the very backbone of the BrainGate.

Remember that the Pycnogenol flavonoids perform better as antioxidants than the anthocyanosides. In contrast, anthocyanosides show superior anti-inflammatory properties. Eating a wide variety of flavonoids provides even greater protection for the BrainGate.

The Brain's Waste-Removal System

The BrainGate manages more activities than just permitting and denying entry. In addition to maintaining the brain's uptake of vital nutrients and items critical to brain function, the BrainGate also employs machinery that converts pollutants and drugs into forms that can be removed by the brain.

We will refer to the brain's waste removal in the same way that city garbage workers dispose of waste. A number of garbage trucks (also called efflux systems) cart waste out of the brain. Certain items like L-dopa (converted in the brain to dopamine) cross the BrainGate and are quickly changed into other products. Converting these compounds not only helps control the buildup of harmful chemicals, it also helps to remove the brain's waste products.

A BrainGate enzyme called monoamine oxidase (MAO) converts old brain messenger waste and pollutants into things that can be loaded into garbage cans and removed from the brain. The BrainGate converts these waste products and pollutants by some of the same systems found in the liver. To balance forming too much of the stimulating brain messengers norepinephrine and epinephrine, reuptake occurs in the nerve cells, and MAO converts them into other products. MAO acts like a double-edged sword, since it can also convert some compounds into neurotoxic chemicals, such as the heroin-like contaminate MPTP, which enters the brain on the dopamine shuttle. MAO converts MPTP into a toxic agent that attacks the power generator of the cell (mitochondria) and causes a disease that is virtually identical to Parkinson's. Pesticide exposure has also been linked to Parkinson's disease.

Water in the Brain: Cerebrospinal Fluid

The inside of your brain contains hollow cavities (ventricles) filled with a fluid called cerebrospinal fluid (CSF). A clear, water-like secretion, CSF originates deep within the brain and acts as a shock absorber for the brain and spinal cord. CSF also provides support, since the brain is buoyant and floats within the CSF. The CSF surrounds the suspended brain and cushions it from shock.

The fluids moving through the brain depend on the material coming through the BrainGate and on removal from the brain by the CSF, which transports waste items into the veins or venous system. Filtered items and compounds originating from the blood make up the CSF. The CSF migrates from the inner brain under pressure and eventually exits the brain into veins like storm gutters. Toxic agents removed by the CSF follow a highly specialized route.

Brain Garbage Trucks: Efflux Proteins

All living cells contain structures called multidrug efflux transporters. The efflux proteins work by helping the cell rid itself of assorted chemicals that otherwise would build up to toxic levels. Therefore, the efflux proteins act like garbage trucks, removing waste products and protecting cells from a buildup of toxic waste. For our purposes, we will refer to the efflux proteins as garbage trucks that are able to drive from inside the brain, through the BrainGate, and then out, dumping their contents in a landfill (the blood vessels).

But this system is a double-edged sword, since it is active in harmful cells, too. Antibiotic-resistant bacteria have been in the news frequently, since they have become a major problem in recent years. Bacteria use their own garbage trucks to establish resistance to antibiotics. Here's how it happens: The bacteria develop efflux proteins that learn how to expel antibiotics from within the cell quicker than the antibiotics can enter the cell. This action renders the antibiotics useless. The bacteria are also known to swap garbage trucks freely, and soon a large population can acquire resistance to antibiotics. A great challenge facing the drug industry is to overcome drug resistance, where brain cells truck the drug out of the brain and disable the effect of the drugs' action.

A number of garbage trucks in the brain collect different toxic compounds and truck them out of the brain. Since the garbage trucks are so broad in their ability to expel so many different substances, their precise operation remains unexplained.

BrainGate garbage trucks have arcane names such as P-glycoprotein (P-gp) and multi-drug resistance-associated protein (MRP). P-gp garbage trucks remove and dump dozens of very dissimilar drugs or toxic agents outside the brain. Of course, the garbage trucks need fuel to drive from the brain to the outside landfill. Anything toxic to the cells' power generator (mitochondria), such as pesticides and heavy metals, like mercury, will eventually cause the garbage trucks to run out of gas.

Studies have shown that the pesticide ivermectin, when given to mice with defective MRP garbage trucks, increases brain levels of the pesticide 80-fold compared with animals with properly working MRP garbage trucks. Toxic agents that decrease the cell's fuel supply will stop the garbage trucks from removing waste and allow a toxic buildup. Thus the brain's sanitation crew is vital for waste removal and continued brain wellness.

3

Red Light

Avoiding the Toxic Agents

OVER ONE TRILLION nerve cells make up the human brain. The nerve cells, or neurons, connect to one another in a complex network. For example, each single neuron attaches to about a thousand other neurons within the brain. So it's not surprising that a number of environmental pollutants that cause nerve cell death can disrupt complex brain functions.

Many modern-day neurotoxic agents have been released into the environment and have exposed people to unprecedented risks. Common sources of neurotoxic agents in the environment range from pesticides used in farming and around the house, to heavy metals like mercury and lead used in paints, to industrial chemicals like PCBs used as insulating fluids in electrical equipment.

Unlike other areas of the body, the brain has only limited ability to regenerate lost cells. The brain contains tissue that is held in reserve for eventual use throughout life. People in industrialized countries over a lifetime slowly but surely deplete their reserve brain tissue until they reach a point where mental decline occurs.

The brain can compensate for some cell death by shifting lost functions to other areas, hiding damage that will eventually reveal itself at more advanced ages. The reserve tissue buffer and the compensating action of the brain complicate the effects of toxicity so that damage may not be expressed until decades following exposure. One can survive exposure to a particular toxic agent and the minor loss of nerve cells that follows and not detect it; however, the same exposure and minor loss continued over decades can result in major brain impairment with advancing age.

While many items have been "linked" to nervous system diseases, they may not have passed the gold standard of scientific proof to be labeled "neurotoxic." Reasons for this uncertainty include the facts that the nervous system may not show damage until decades after the toxic exposure and that research is limited by the ethical limits of experimenting on humans.

Humans possess one of the most sophisticated brains on the planet, certainly much different from a rat's brain. Yet animal studies alone form the basis for many decisions regarding chemical use. Countless items confront modern people every day with potential risks to brain health and function. In addition, many neurotoxic agents combined in low doses may show significant toxicity even though they show little when given alone. Unfortunately, we do not have sufficient human toxicity data even on individual neurotoxic agents. Studying the combined effects of different mixtures of neurotoxic items in the environment would prove extremely costly. Absolute scientific proof will, therefore, not arrive soon, since exposure occurs more or less to everyone and we no longer have unexposed control groups for comparison. And because ethical constraints prohibit human experiments that cause serious damage to health, we must operate with incomplete data in the future.

The Ten Most Powerful Neurotoxic Foods

1. High-chemical-input commercial produce (laden with pesticides, many of which are neurotoxic)
2. Neurotoxic food contaminates, especially concentrated in animal product foods (organochlorines like PCBs and dioxin)
3. Fried, high-fat foods (oxidized fats, acrylamide)
4. Overprocessed foods, especially those with hydrogenated oils (trans-fatty acids)
5. Seafood, especially predatory fish like shark, swordfish, and trout (methylmercury, PCBs), and fugu fish (Japan) (tetrodotoxin)
6. Shellfish (trimethyltin, cadmium, domoic acid, saxitoxin, and ciguatera toxin)
7. Neurotoxic food additives (aspartame [NutraSweet], monosodium glutamate [MSG])
8. Potatoes, especially those left in sunlight that have turned green (glycoalkaloids such as solanine)
9. Supplements (some calcium supplements have high levels of neurotoxic lead)
10. Highly processed foods like cheese, over-the-counter antacids like Mylanta and Rolaids, nondairy creamers, table salt, and baking soda (can have high levels of neurotoxic aluminum)

Common Metal Pollutants

Let's imagine for a moment that societies around the globe decide not to release any toxic chemicals into the environment. Many people might be led to believe that this novel policy could return our planet shortly to its pristine state. But would it? Unfortunately, metals such as cadmium, lead, and mercury tenaciously persist in our environment. Automobiles and industry have caused more than a 300-fold increase in lead levels measured in Greenland ice, since 880 B.C. Nature treats many human-made pollutants as foreign and degrades them slowly or not at all. Many environmental pollutants harm the brain.

Therefore, for healthy existence in a modern world with a contaminated food supply, humans need to alter their diets. You must limit foods that contain persistent pollutants, which can collect in your body from cradle to grave. Persistent poisons include the metals cadmium, lead, and (to a smaller degree) mercury and the organochlorine chemicals like dioxin, PCB, and DDT. Lead dulls IQ, cadmium causes kidney disorders, and mercury is toxic to the nervous system. These effects appear to be irreversible.

Lead Levels Found in the Greenland Ice Cap

Lead Level*	Era
0.5	880 B.C.
2–3	500 B.C. to 300 A.D. (Generated by Greek and Roman smeltring)
4	Middle Ages and Renaissance
10	Industrial Revolution
50	Nineteenth century
100	1960s (200 times the estimated natural value)
150	1984 (300 times the estimated natural value; attributed to lead additives in gasoline)

**in picograms of lead per gram of ice*

Lead

It has been speculated that the harmful effects of lead such as low birth weight, increased childhood mortality, and psychiatric disorders in the ruling class may have played a role in the decline of the

Roman Empire. Rome's ruling class contaminated itself with the use of lead materials in aqueducts and food vessels. In modern times the use of lead-based paints and fuel has contaminated much of the globe.

Lead Passes Through the BrainGate

Toxic lead crosses the BrainGate and may cause senile dementia and Alzheimer's. More recently, lead has been linked with learning disabilities such as attention-deficit disorder and various aggressive behaviors. Lead poisoning impacts the prefrontal cortex, which governs impulse behavior and may cause one to react violently if disrupted. The lasting side effects from lead poisoning build up, and the toxic effects can persist over a lifetime.

Lead can damage the capillaries that make up the BrainGate and harm the glial cells that nurture nerve cells. Lead disrupts calcium and various brain messengers critical for controlling emotions, learning, and memory. For example, lead blocks the formation of dopamine and serotonin. Mental functions such as impulse control and managing violent behaviors depend on dopamine and serotonin. At least seven studies have shown that violent criminals have elevated levels of lead, cadmium, manganese, mercury, and other toxins compared with prisoners who were not violent. Lead also produces a progressive mental decline.

Most studies show that dietary lead is poorly absorbed and that adults retain about 5 to 15 percent of it. Children, however, can absorb over 40 percent of lead. Once absorbed, lead eventually travels to the bones and stays for decades or longer. Infants and children in a rapid growth phase absorb more metals such as lead than adults do. Milk also increases lead and cadmium absorption. Casein, a primary milk protein, has also demonstrated an ability to increase lead levels in the brain, liver, and kidneys of animals, compared with animals that received a soybean diet. A diet containing soybeans actually reduced lead absorption and toxicity. The high fat content of milk also enhances lead and environmental pollutant uptake. Elevating the dietary fat of animals from 5 to 20 percent doubled the level of lead detected in the blood. Saturated butterfat showed the most dramatic increase in lead uptake, while polyunsaturated sunflower oils had a small effect on lead uptake. The primary milk sugar, lactose, also enables greater absorption of lead when compared with other dietary sugars.

By contrast, the fruit sugar pectin bound up lead and decreased its uptake. In addition, industrial lead workers showed increased lead removal when their diet contained a large amount of carrots and cabbage.

Foods high in fruit pectin (apples are a good source) and in the sulfur amino acids methionine and cysteine (such as garlic, onions, and beans) have been found to increase lead removal. Sweating assists a little in lead and environmental pollutant removal. Since lead competes with calcium for absorption, calcium-rich foods block lead uptake. Foods high in calcium include oranges, spinach, rhubarb, collards, dried figs, turnips, kale, okra, tofu (or soybeans), white beans, pinto beans, baked beans, and broccoli.

Sources of Lead Exposure

Colored glossy newsprint, soil, and water all contain lead. Rice and vegetables cooked in lead-contaminated water will absorb 80 percent of the lead. Some canned foods can contain lead. Food wrapping can contain lead, and sometimes the grinding of meat will increase its lead content. The plastic insulation of wires often contains lead. Houses built before 1980 usually contain lead-based paints. While estimates vary, 60 to 80 percent of homes built before 1980 are thought to have used lead-based paint. The greatest source of global lead pollution, however, resulted from the use of leaded gasoline. Other sources of lead include candlewicks and burning candles, which can result in higher levels of lead in the air of homes. Many of the imported vinyl mini-blinds used lead-containing additives for greater strength and color stability. Tests have confirmed that the dust released from vinyl mini-blinds contains high levels of lead. Do not use calcium supplements especially ones using bonemeals since they also contain lead (see Appendix).

Mercury

Bacteria convert mercury into a form called methylmercury that enters the food chain. Fish and seafood harbor the most easily absorbed form of methylmercury. Predatory fish contain the highest amounts of this toxic substance. Fish store methylmercury in the muscle or edible tissues. Mercury does not stay in your body for decades, yet it can quickly build up to toxic levels because it is absorbed over 90 percent from foods.

Mercury's Link to Alzheimer's Disease

People with Alzheimer's disease have blood levels of mercury three times higher than people who don't have Alzheimer's. Research has shown that mercury has toxic effects on cultured nerve cells. By adding very low levels of mercury to cultured neurons, researchers found seven characteristic cell features that typify Alzheimer's disease. While this finding does not prove mercury can cause Alzheimer's, we do know that mercury clearly causes toxicity to the brain.

Sources of Mercury Exposure

We need to limit or eliminate the amount of seafood we consume, especially fish that prey on other fish. Predatory fish such as shark, swordfish, pike, and barracuda (any fish with teeth) will have much higher levels of mercury and PCB. Deep-ocean halibut and flounder have fewer pollutants. Freshwater fish tend to harbor higher amounts of mercury.

Vaccines also use mercury-based preservatives. A mercury-based chemical called thimerosal is used as a preservative and suspension agent in many vaccines for adults and children, including infants. Currently a hotly contested debate links mercury-preserved vaccines to autism and other learning disorders in children. Therefore, make sure your health clinic uses mercury-free flu vaccines. Ask to see the package insert that comes shipped with the flu vaccines and look for the presence of thimerosal preservatives.

Cadmium

Cadmium is a metal used in batteries and electronic circuits. Sewage sludge contains high levels of cadmium and is now used to fertilize commercial crops but not organic crops. Studies in Sweden demonstrate a slow and steady increase in cadmium content that has occurred in crops over time. For most people cadmium exposure comes from eating contaminated foods.

Sources of Cadmium Exposure

Filter-feeding shellfish like mussels, oysters, shrimp, crab, snails, and fish also tend to have high amounts of cadmium. Shellfish are exposed to cadmium from the water and then accumulate it by attaching it to cadmium-binding proteins.

Cadmium is also found in cereal grains, root crops, and leafy vegetables. Plants readily take up cadmium more than other metals. Cadmium can pollute soil through fallout from air and from commercial fertilizers or irrigation water. Cadmium, although not very well absorbed (5 to 8 percent) from the diet, also sets up camp in the human body for decades. Organ meats like liver, and especially kidney, can contain high levels of cadmium. Soft tissues, especially the kidney, progressively store cadmium, and this accumulation correlates well with the onset of chronic disease.

Cigarettes are another source of cadmium—smoking one pack a day might double your daily absorbed burden of cadmium.

Be careful choosing zinc supplements, since some are contaminated with cadmium. Cadmium is absorbed from drinking water more easily than from other dietary sources. Plant fibers can reduce cadmium absorption. Plant products like lignan and cellulose dramatically reduce cadmium uptake.

Aluminum

Aluminum is the most abundant metal found in the earth's crust. Until fairly recently, aluminum existed mostly in forms not absorbed by people and other animals. But this changed with the development of acid rain, which allowed aluminum uptake in food chains. Aluminum released from acid rain damages fish gills and eventually kills fish in acid-dead lakes.

Aluminum toxicity in animals first appears as subtle behavioral changes such as decreased learning and memory functions. Aluminum causes the most common early tissue buildup of neurofibrillary tangles or NFTs. NFTs are twisted and tangled filaments found within nerve cells. They have been found especially in the cerebral cortex and hippocampus in the brains of Alzheimer's patients. Not all species show NFTs—rats don't, but monkeys and humans do.

O

Foods High in Aluminum

—Beverages in aluminum cans
—Processed cereals such as Post Raisin Bran
—Baking sodas and powders
—Iodized salt and table salt
—Nondairy creamers such as Coffeemate
—Processed cheese such as Kraft, Cracker Barrel
—Gelatin desserts, Jell-O
—Processed cookies such as Oreos
—Canned vegetables
—Baby formulas

People who undergo kidney dialysis sometimes show a fatal brain syndrome. The patients have higher aluminum content in the brain and first show speech disorders and then dementia. The source of the elevated aluminum levels is the oral aluminum compounds given or the aluminum used in the dialysis fluid.

Aluminum and Alzheimer's Disease

The connections between aluminum and Alzheimer's have been hotly debated for decades. The debate began when researchers found increased aluminum content in the brains of people suffering from Alzheimer's. Some contend that elevated aluminum results from a leaky BrainGate that simply allows more aluminum into the brain. As we age, the BrainGate can become less protective and allow more aluminum across. Currently the precise role of aluminum in causing Alzheimer's is not known, yet we do know that aluminum can exert neurotoxic effects and that our exposure to aluminum should be minimized.

Sources of Aluminum Exposure

Many pharmaceutical drugs use aluminum-containing binding agents, and antacids like Mylanta, Remegel, Rolaids, and Pepto-Bismol contain very high amounts of aluminum. Many vitamin supplements such as vitamin C use silica-binding agents that contain aluminum. Unfiltered drinking water can also contain aluminum. Cooking in aluminum pots and pans can transfer aluminum to food.

Environmental Pollutants

Most people accept declines in cognitive ability as they grow older as part of the normal aging process. But some mental decline may result from prior exposures to neurotoxic agents. By being aware of proper diet and lifestyle, we can prevent some progressive mental decline.

Environmental chemicals use a number of routes to gain access to your body. Most enter through your mouth and some get inhaled or absorbed by the skin. How do we accelerate the removal of neurotoxic environmental chemicals? The liver processes most of the diet as well as environmental chemicals. Unfortunately, during the process of removing chemicals, the liver can also change some non-toxic chemicals into toxic ones. Polycyclic aromatic hydrocarbons (PAHs), a class of chemicals metabolized into more toxic versions, can also form with high-temperature food processing.

The liver changes chemicals with long resident times such as benzene into forms that can dissolve in water and be passed in the urine. Therefore, the kidneys act as another toxic removal organ. The kidney transfers smaller-sized chemicals chemicals into the urine. Generous water intake maintains a continuous removal of many environmental chemicals. By drinking sufficient amounts of water, you remove many chemicals before they can build up to neurotoxic levels.

The liver and kidneys play vital roles in the changing balance between the amount of environmental pollutants that is stored in the body and the amount that's removed. When the balance shifts toward storage, your brain can suffer damage. The two main routes for pollutants to exit are in urine and feces.

Substances that dissolve in fats can be stored in fat deposits, where they can persist for years. Think about the way vinegar and oil do not stay mixed and need a vigorous shake before using. Vinegar acts more like water and will not mix with the oil. Similarly, in order to remove the excess fat-soluble items, the liver converts them into compounds that dissolve in water so they can pass out of the body in urine. The liver also makes bile, a dark green substance that is excreted into the small intestine. Bile acts very much like soap by keeping the fats soluble, dissolved in a watery environment. A high-fat meal will trigger a large release of bile, assisting in the gut's uptake of fat.

The liver rids the body of items by attaching various sugars to the fat-soluble compounds that assist in the removal. Plant chemicals found in such foods as cabbage, broccoli, and cauliflower increase the activity of certain enzymes and help in the removal processes.

The bile attaches and binds up environmental chemicals, but when these materials travel down to the large intestine, certain bacteria can act on them and release them back as fat-soluble items, allowing reuptake. This removal and reuptake becomes a toxic cycle that increases the time necessary to clear pollutants from the body and leads to chemical persistence.

To break this cycle of persistence, plant fiber can attach to the bile complexes and remove them together through feces. The constant removal of bile complexes not only decreases the uptake of environmental chemicals, it also lessens their toxicity.

Plant-based diets help to maintain a healthy brain in another way as well. A number of neurotoxic compounds attach to bile, including arsenic, cadmium, lead, manganese, mercury, DDT, and PCB. It's a matter of choice: eat a plant-rich diet and neurotoxic compounds will travel into the sewage system instead of being stored in your body. Plant fiber also speeds food through the gut, thus reducing the risk of a leaky gut and many intestinal disorders.

The two basic types of dietary fiber are soluble and insoluble forms. Soluble fibers can dissolve in water and produce a gel-like substance. Apples, grapefruit, and grains such as oat and psyllium contain soluble fibers. On the other hand, insoluble fiber undergoes minimal changes in the intestine and passes out largely unchanged. Insoluble fibers are found in bran cereals, whole wheat, and rice bran. Industrial food processing largely removes the fiber or degrades it to a finely ground form, which doesn't provide the same protection as do coarse fibers or the fibers found in whole plant foods.

The large intestine has some of the most densely populated bacteria in the gut. Food plays an important role in providing specific nutrients to intestinal microbes. The gut bacteria convert environmental chemicals when they pass through the intestine. A high-fiber diet will speed the gut's removal of pollutants and decrease the bacterial conversion of pollutants. Mercury can be dramatically recycled in bile and reabsorbed into the body by the gut. Wheat bran not only decreases the uptake of mercury by 30 percent but it also eliminates this poison from the body up to 43 percent faster. A recent study showed that rice bran and spinach fiber removed the pollutant PCB. Rice and spinach fibers caused a dramatic increase in PCB removal from the body (4.1 to 6.6 times greater removal). A brain-healthy diet needs to include these indispensable plant fibers.

Reducing Neurotoxic Pollutant Loads

There are many avenues you can take to cut down on your exposure to brain-damaging chemical pollutants. Making simple changes in what you eat and drink and some simple adjustments in how you live can help keep you—and your brain—out of harm's way.

Eat More Plants

Organic vegetables and fruits contain fewer amounts of neurotoxic pesticides and heavy metals. Plant fiber blocks gut tumor formation.

Insoluble, coarse fiber that does not dissolve and form a gel is more consistent in blocking cancer. Plant fibers reduce food passage time through the gut, help to condition the gut, prevent a leaky gut, and reduce the formation of toxic secondary bile acids.

Drink More Purified Water

Drink generous amounts of filtered water, which will increase removal of chemicals through urine. Don't drink tap water or beverages made from tap water.

Eat Fewer Animal Products

For millennia domesticated animals have provided a high-protein source in the form of meat and dairy products. However, because of today's animal-product-based livestock feed, changing practices in farming, and increasing industrialization, our meat, poultry, fish, and dairy products are now responsible for about 60 to 80 percent of the pesticide and organochlorine chemical residues in the American diet.

The organochlorine pollutants—a class of industrial chemicals that have been widely dumped into our environment—include dioxin, PCBs, and pesticides, which are toxic to the brain and depress the immune system. Some organochlorines quite easily cross into the brain and kill brain cells. PCBs and dioxin in particular can also interrupt the chemical and electrical communication within the brain. PCBs, for example, can affect learning by blocking the brain messenger dopamine. Animal products do not contain the pollutant-removing fibers that plants have in such abundance.

After you consume a meal of mostly animal products, fat saturates the blood, which becomes thick like sludge, thereby increasing the chance of a blood clot. Another peril of eating red meat is too much iron. Advertisers are forever urging us to get enough iron in our diet. Yet who thinks about the toxic consequences of excess iron? Red meat contains heme iron, a form of iron that is very effectively absorbed. Few people realize the toxic effects of high iron storage, which causes increased heart disease and senile dementia. During their reproductive years, women shed iron in their monthly menstrual cycle. In contrast, men cannot remove iron unless they donate blood, making them more prone to heart disease and dementia. After menopause, a woman's risk for heart disease is similar to that for a man. And a recent study in Sweden showed a reduction in cancer risk in blood donors.

The brain starts to accumulate more iron with advancing age. Most people with major brain diseases, such as Parkinson's disease, Alzheimer's dementia, and amyotrophic lateral sclerosis (ALS, or Lou Gehrig's disease) show elevated iron levels. Iron and copper can accelerate the formation of free radicals. In addition, as we get older, we make less of the iron transport protein (transferrin) that attaches to free iron and ferries iron in the blood. Because of this, older people have less ability to process iron. If you continue to eat large portions of red meat, you will likely have higher levels of iron in your blood, tissues, and brain. Free iron harms the brain, since it can increase free radicals and destroy structural fats. Eating excess red meat can also lead to increased brain disease, cancer, and heart disease risk. Recently, a German study has linked the high intake of meat and organ meat (kidney and liver) to increased rates of Parkinson's disease. Other studies have linked high intakes of red meat to increased incidence of senile dementia.

Meat Is Bad for the Brain

—Contains high amounts of saturated fats—which cause heart and vessel diseases—and contains the largest dietary source of environmental pollutants.

—Causes protein overload. Excess protein may cause leaky gut syndrome, which affects brain health, and leads to other severe medical conditions such as kidney stones.

—Causes sodium overload. Meat is high in sodium, which can lead to high blood pressure, a condition that negatively affects brain health.

—Causes iron overload. Iron from red meat is easily absorbed and can cause heart disease and cancer. High intakes of red meat have been linked to increased brain iron and senile dementia.

—Contains neurotoxic and immune system poisons, such as heavy metals, dioxin, and PCBs.

—Contains excess arachidonic acid, which is turned into prostaglandins, causing inflammation that can affect the BrainGate.

Avoid or Limit Processed Foods

One of the food industry's primary goals is to extend the shelf life of processed foods. Even one more day of shelf life will increase profits.

Some highly processed foods have very long shelf lives. Processed foods also include those fancy nutrition bars, which are simply candy bars with added vitamins. Most processed foods contain hydrolyzed proteins, a method food makers use to hide potentially neurotoxic flavor enhancers, since food labels don't list glutamate and aspartate as ingredients. Stay away from foods that contain MSG, hydrolyzed proteins, and similar types of additives.

Many processed foods contain high amounts of calories, but those are empty calories (calories from sugar and fat), stripped of nutritious agents. Highly processed canned foods lack nutrition and most contain high levels of salt and many potentially neurotoxic food additives.

Most processed foods have destroyed foods' inherent critical nutrients and fats through grinding, overheating, and chemical bleaching. For example, bleached white flour fed to rats did not provide enough nutrition for their survival. Because of this lack of nutritional value the FDA required the bleached-flour makers to add vitamins to processed flour. The food purveyors then started calling bleached flour *enriched* flour! Remember, if the food label does not state specifically that the product contains "unbleached flour," then it contains bleached flour.

Many processed foods contain partially hydrogenated vegetable oils that cause heart disease and harm your general health and brain functions. As explained earlier, food processors hydrogenate oils by heating them to extreme temperatures, adding a metal catalyst, and bubbling hydrogen gas through the oil to form unnatural trans-fats. Many human studies show the toxicity of trans-fats, found in processed food such as margarine and shortenings. Trans-fats–rich diets will likely lead to neurotoxicity, cancer, and heart disease.

The food industry adds hydrogenated oils to a variety of products because they impart a desirable texture and creaminess and greatly increase the shelf life of processed foods. But be sure to read the ingredient list of every product you purchase, since the current label laws do not require disclosure of the amount of trans-fats contained in any given food. Food makers only list the total fat and saturated fat contents of foods. Avoid all foods that contain margarine or any oil that is partially hydrogenated or hydrogenated.

Eliminate fried foods from your diet, too. You brain won't do well with fried foods. The high temperatures needed to fry foods actually break down fats, or oxidize them, in a process that is similar to that of butter turning rancid. French fries and other fried foods contain the neurotoxic compound called acrylamide. The high-temperature frying not only introduces rancid fats, it also destroys critical vitamins like E and C. Diets high in oxidized fats also lead to strange foam cells that appear in the bloodstream. Foam cells play a critical role in the process of heart disease, cancer, and, ultimately, reduced mental functioning.

For most people, diet is the most critical intake route for environmental chemicals. Since many pollutants persist in the body, you need to decrease your exposure to them. The persistent chemicals like PCBs, cadmium, and lead can be greatly avoided by limiting your intake of dairy and other animal products.

A brain-enhancing nutrition plan also removes all processed food from the diet, including but not limited to packaged meats (bologna and hot dogs) instant potatoes, canned goods, snacks, cakes, and frozen dinners. Read the food labels and if they contain more

Processed Food: Unhealthy for the Brain

— Processed food contains very high levels of simple sugars that cause decreased mental acuity when blood glucose levels fall.

— Processed food is loaded with neurotoxic additives like tran-fats and acrylamide.

— Processing strips anti-cancer agents, antioxidants, and minerals like glutathione that cannot be obtained from any other source in your diet.

— Artificial sweeteners disrupt amino acid uptake in the brain and may cause toxicity and hyperactivity in children.

— Artificial dyes have been linked to hyperactivity in children.

— Bleached flour lacks nutrition and contains unnatural products.

— Toxic products like the cancer-causing heterocyclic amines are formed by high-heat processing.

— Processing forms unnatural toxic amino acids that disrupt DNA manufacture.

— Pollutant-removing plant fiber is degraded and removed from many food products during processing.

— Processed foods have high levels of trans-fatty acids and other oxidized fats that are linked to heart disease and cancer.

— Processed foods contain abnormally high levels of salt, which leads to high blood pressure and contains brain-toxic aluminum.

than five ingredients, don't purchase them. Nutritious food sources are listed in the Appendix.

Pesticides

When people established agricultural settlements they began looking for ways to protect their crops. Early farmers used sulfur to guard crops from insects long before 500 B.C. Toxic formulations of lead, arsenic, and mercury protected crops from pests in the 1400s. In the 1600s nicotine compounds from tobacco leaves served as pesticides. By the middle 1800s, farmers extracted the heads of chrysanthemum flowers to isolate pyrethrum and rotenone from the derris plant. While first-generation pesticides mostly originated from plants, chemistry labs gave birth to the second-generation pesticides such as DDT. A major chemical industry sprang up after the discovery of the potent insect-killing properties of DDT by entomologist Paul Müller. DDT soon became the planet's most popular pesticide and, ironically, Müller received the Nobel Prize in 1948 for his discovery.

In the 1930s the United States had crop yields similar to those of India, England, and Argentina. Since the 1950s the use of petroleum-derived pesticides, fertilizers, and a host of governmental policies have vaulted the United States into position as the biggest farming economy in the world. Today, fewer farmers feed more people than ever before in the history of food production. This farming success, however, has not occurred without enormous costs and environmental tradeoffs.

Pesticide proponents argue that the benefits of their poisons far outweigh their harm. After all, pesticides do save lives. Since the late 1940s, DDT has prevented millions from contracting malaria, bubonic plague, and typhus. Proponents also contend that pesticides work faster and more effectively than the alternatives. Pesticide advocates also point out that the new-generation pesticides, when used at very low application rates, decrease human exposure compared with the outdated products. Today the world uses about 2.5

million tons of pesticides yearly. Cultivation of just four crops—soybeans, wheat, cotton, and corn—consumes approximately 75 percent of the pesticides in the United States.

Every day, the environmental and health consequences of commercial farming become more apparent. Insects breed rapidly and quickly develop resistance to pesticides. In addition, broad-spectrum pesticides also kill natural predators that keep pests in check. Synthetic pesticide use has increased more than 33-fold in the last half-century. Ironically, more of the U.S. food supply is lost to pests today (37 percent) than in the 1940s (31 percent).

Experts have also shown that pesticide application does not guarantee increased crop yields. According to David Pimentel, professor of Insect Ecology and Agricultural Sciences at Cornell University, "Although pesticides are generally profitable, their use does not always decrease crop losses. For example, even with the 10-fold increase in insecticide use in the United States from 1945 to 1989, total crop losses from insect damage have nearly doubled from 7 percent to 13 percent."

In addition, as farmers have become addicted to pesticides, animal production has gotten hooked on antibiotics. For more than 40 years, ranchers and animal growers have been feeding low levels of penicillin, tetracycline, and other antibiotics to poultry, cattle, and pigs to speed growth and cut costs. That use accounts for about one-third to one-half of all antibiotics sold in the United States. Scientists worldwide

Reducing Neurotoxin Exposure Around the House

—Air out your dry-cleaned clothes before you wear them or bring them indoors. Request paper bags, not plastic, to cover your dry-cleaned clothes.

—Use Pür-brand water filters or install a reverse-osmosis unit in your house.

—Use HEPA filters at home on the furnace. Use particulate filters on the house windows.

—Keep your home free from neurotoxic pesticides (see Appendix).

—Don't use aluminum and plastic in cooking (see Appendix).

—Make sure your home is lead-free (see Appendix).

—Peel or wash commercial produce or use a special soap (see Appendix).

—Be cautious of hobby materials that use lead, such as stained glass, billiard chalks, and ceramics.

—Replace plastic mini-blinds with wood or metal blinds.

have criticized the use of antibiotics to promote animal growth because it increases the prevalence of bacteria resistant to antibiotics and jeopardizes human health.

Pesticides and nitrates from fertilizers and manure have been detected in the groundwater of almost every state in the nation. In fact, scientists have measured pollutants from agriculture in both the North and South Poles and in the deepest reaches of the oceans. Most food available has detectable levels of pesticides and antibiotics. In recent studies these same substances have been implicated as possible culprits in causing Parkinson's disease as well as increased aggression in children. Furthermore, in 1998, the EPA reported agriculture as the single largest nonpoint polluter of our rivers and streams, fouling more than 173,000 miles of waterways with chemicals, erosion, and animal waste from raising livestock. Aside from the animal-waste runoff, a good share of this chemical pollution results from growing livestock and feeds using chemically dependent agriculture. Today, pesticides have been measured in the fat and body tissues of all human groups on the planet except for a select group of Indian tribes living deep in the Amazon jungle.

Recent studies show that trace levels of multiple pesticides cause increased aggression. Aggression in humans was triggered with trace combinations of pesticides, but not with exposure to a single pesticide. Specifically, trace pesticide mixtures are associated with abnormally increased thyroid hormone levels. Irritability, aggression, and multiple chemical sensitivity are all associated with thyroid hormone levels. Also, compounds such as nitrates (converted into cancer-producing chemicals) have become more prevalent in commercially grown produce because of the overuse of nitrogen-containing fertilizers.

Brain-Healthy Reasons to Eat Organic Foods

Commercially grown crops fertilized with concentrated nitrates contain high levels of nitrates that are converted into toxic nitrosamines when eaten. Nitrosamines are linked to brain and other cancers. Although manure used in organic farming also contains nitrates, this source does not migrate to the ground water as quickly as does commercial fertilizer.

Many health benefits come from eating organically grown produce. One major difference between organic and high-chemical-input food lies in the use of pesticides and commercial fertilizers. Commercially grown fruits and vegetables will often have multiple pesticide residues. Commercially grown strawberries alone, for example, can contain over sixty different pesticides.

Unlike organic produce, grown using rotation of the soil plots and careful stewardship of the soil, commercially grown crops deplete the soil nutrients by repeated growth in the same soil plots. What the plant can't obtain from the depleted soil it gets from the overuse of fertilizer. High-chemical-input crops have become completely dependent upon the use of fertilizers and pesticides, and the sterilized soil virtually serves only to hold the crops in place.

By contrast, organic farms have much higher concentrations of life-giving organic matter in the soil. A soil high in organic matter provides more water-holding capacities and, therefore, improves drought tolerance and reduces the activity and migration of pesticides. Further, organic matter in soil serves as a depot for select nutrients and assists in keeping these nutrients available. Organically grown produce has been shown to have up to three times more minerals and trace elements than commercially grown produce.

There have been conflicting studies on the ultimate nutritional value of organic produce. Some studies show organic food provides more nutrition than commercially grown, whereas others claim that organic foods have the same nutritional value as commercial produce. Unfortunately, far more research has been directed to aid mechanized, commercial agriculture in producing foods of uniform size and uniform dates of ripening. Commercial agriculture, with its focus on mechanical harvesting and large-scale storage, transport, and processing, also consumes vast quantities of energy in the form of oil, gas, and electricity. Organic farming does not rely on the intensive use of inputs such as chemical fertilizers and pesticides. Instead it relies on natural soil builders and biological control of pests. Organic farming uses much less energy than commercial farming and therefore generates fewer greenhouse gases, such as carbon dioxide.

Just about any consumer can note the difference between an organically grown tomato and a commercially grown tomato. The organic tomato has a rich, deep red color that indicates the presence of the red pigment lycopene, a health-protective plant chemical known to help reduce lung and prostate cancers. Commercial growers pick green tomatoes and ship them to receiving stations that use ethylene oxide gas to force them to ripen. Tomatoes treated in this manner will often have much lower lycopene levels. Recent studies also show that organic produce contains more healthy plant chemicals called phytochemicals. Many of these phytochemicals such as lycopene (in tomatoes) and resveratrol (in grapes) have been linked to reduced heart disease and cancer risk.

The Effects of Pesticide Exposure

The diet serves as the most significant route for exposure, especially if you do not farm or work in the chemical industry. Home and garden application of pesticides can expose many people through skin contact, inhalation, and ingestion, and by infiltration into food and water.

By design, pesticides destroy or slow the growth of undesirable forms of insect, plant, animal, or fungal life. In fact, some herbicides kill plants by attacking the power generator of the cell—the mitochondria. Plant and animal mitochondria share similar features; therefore, herbicides may harm human mitochondria. When herbicides poison the mitochondria, these power generators cannot produce energy, which in turn may harm the brain cells.

Pesticides have the puzzling ability to show "delayed neurotoxic effects." The toxic effect to the brain often does not surface until many years after exposure. The most common causes of accidental poisonings involve organophosphate and carbamate pesticides that can show toxicity years after a single exposure. Malathion, an organophosphate pesticide, can irreversibly damage the nervous system following a single large exposure. Most brain and nervous system deficits will surface much later in life, and this delay complicates full identification of cause-and-effect relationships. For example, memory impairment, dementia, or Alzheimer's disease may result from a large chemical exposure that occurred early in life or from small daily exposures to neurotoxic agents over time.

Usually the levels of pesticides in tissues with high fat content may be 100 to 300 times greater than in the bloodstream. Since the brain contains large amounts of fat, it's not unexpected that behavioral changes like memory declines, emotional disturbances, depression, and lack of concentration have become sensitive indicators of exposure to fat-soluble pesticides. Pesticides can impede concentration, increase learning disabilities, decrease memory, and cause aggression, mood swings, and other neurological symptoms.

Other research shows that human exposure to very small levels of certain pesticides can change brain function enough to cause prolonged periods of insomnia, irritability, loss of libido, and decreased concentration. The most sensitive indicators of pesticide exposure include emotional imbalance and memory problems such as recalling names and words. Farm workers exposed to pesticides display mental declines and higher incidences of Parkinson's disease than nonfarmers.

Food Additives

Commercially prepared foods are loaded with "flavor enhancers," "stabilizers," and other chemical additives used to make food taste better and have better "mouth-feel," and to extend shelf life. These additives, especially glutamate, aspartate, and MSG, are all known excitotoxins, meaning they literally excite cells to the point of death.

Excitotoxins interact with receptors and overexcite nerve cells, leading to the death of brain cells. Excitotoxic agents are linked to brain diseases such as Alzheimer's, Parkinson's, and ALS. Scientists also believe that excitotoxicity can cause age-related memory loss, confusion, and mental decline.

As discussed in Chapter 2, a number of brain messengers stimulate and regulate the brain's vital operations. For example, the brain uses the amino acids glutamate and aspartate as the primary excitatory brain messengers.

Brain messengers allow brain cells to communicate with each other. Brain messengers can either excite nerve cells to fire an electrical current on their surfaces, or inhibit them. Brain messengers remain inside the nerve cells in small, bubble-like structures called vesicles and, when released, they migrate to the receiving nerve cells. If enough brain messengers reach the nerve cell, it will fire an electrical current in response.

Glutamate and aspartate are the most common excitotoxic amino acids. Glutamate directs nerves messages to respond to sensations of taste and hearing as well as thinking and memory. Because of the wide-ranging functions of glutamate and aspartate, the human brain transports and stores them. In very minute concentrations (approximately 10-millionths of a gram) glutamate functions as a brain messenger. However, when glutamate levels outside the nerve cell rise higher, the nerves start to fire erratically. If glutamate rises even more, the nerves are excited to the point of death (or excitotoxicity). Further, nerve cells in a low energy state enhance the excitotoxicity response.

Sources of Food Additives and Excitotoxic Agents

A variety of processed foods commonly contain the flavor enhancer MSG (monosodium glutamate). All sorts of foods, from soups and gravies to potato chips and crackers, all can contain MSG. In particular, low-calorie or diet foods contain large amounts of flavor enhancers with excitotoxic potential. Many canned and processed soups and gravies typically contain multiple types of excitotoxic additives such as hydrolyzed proteins. Hydrolyzed proteins contain high levels of glutamate and other flavor enhancers. Soups or liquid foods flood into the bloodstream quickly and can display even more excitotoxicity. Wheat gluten contains over 40 percent glutamate; casein, the primary milk protein, is 23 percent glutamate; and beef gelatin protein is 12 percent glutamate. Red meat, processed tomatoes, and cheeses are also known to contain high levels of glutamate.

The artificial sweetener aspartame (NutraSweet®) contains 50 percent aspartate, an excitatory amino acid. Aspartame is almost universally present in sugarless chewing gums and desserts, and low-calorie soft drinks. The consumer needs to be wary of food additives since our food processors have disguised additives or free amino acids that have excitotoxic potential with names like hydrolyzed vegetable protein, chicken broth, textured vegetable proteins, hydrolyzed plant proteins, soy extracts, casein or caseinate (a milk protein), yeast extracts, spices, and natural flavors.

The major purveyors of MSG and aspartame use claims about BrainGate function in defense of their product's safety. They claim that the BrainGate excludes these food additives from the brain. But their evidence is not convincing. Multiple doses of food additives can indeed elevate levels of glutamate or aspartate in the brain. Further research has also shown that high levels of glutamate can decrease the amount of glucose entering the brain. Glutamate treatment caused a dramatic (64 percent) reduction in brain glucose. This decline in available energy could work in concert with glutamate to promote excitotoxicity.

Commercial food processors also make the claim that these additives are normal constituents of food—so they must be safe and should be of no concern. However, high levels of free amino acids in foods never challenged humans until the last 50 years. Humans, until recently, have mostly consumed whole foods. Whole foods release their amino acids gradually. Think of this like a time-release capsule, yet sodas or soups do not require digestion and they rapidly flood into the bloodstream and swarm the BrainGate.

A classic example of excitotoxic poisoning occurred in 1987 on Canada's Prince Edward Island, when people consumed domoic acid-contaminated blue mussels. The victims suffered from typical food poisoning symptoms and can vividly recall the details. However, some of the victims would have a difficult time recalling what they ate for breakfast today. Five years after eating the tainted mussels, many of the poisoned have great difficulty recalling things from short-term memory. Short-term memory—the most vulnerable to damage—declines first in advancing age. Does short-term memory decline from a lifetime of eating excitotoxins contained in the processed-food diets of Western nations?

Avoiding Excitotoxicity

The best way to prevent excitotoxicity is to not eat processed foods that contain MSG, hydrolyzed vegetable proteins, and aspartame, and to limit your consumption of shellfish. It's also important to consume a basic antioxidant diet to deter the long-term brain diseases that can result from excitotoxicity. Two important antioxidants are vitamins C and E, since some areas of the brain concentrate vitamin C 10 to 100 times higher than in blood levels. Vitamin E helps to maintain vitamin C in an active form. Vitamin C also plays a central role in the formation of dopamine.

To receive optimal benefits, consume a medley of antioxidants together. If you only consume whole fresh foods, you don't have to worry, since whole food contains a number of vitamins and antioxidant components. Flavonoids from plant pigments are excellent sources of antioxidants for the brain. These food-source antioxidants include polyphenols (blueberries), quercetin (apples, onions, and tea), curcumin (turmeric), rosemary, green tea, ginger, oregano, naringenin (grapefruits), and hesperetin (citrus fruits).

Flavonoids interrupt and block the toxic processes of free radicals. Flavonoids also tie up (or chelate) iron and copper, and they will not make you iron- or copper-deficient. Flavonoids have another amazing benefit: they can aid in repairing and decreasing capillary leakage and actually strengthen the BrainGate. The vital importance of flavonoids in the diet once again stresses the critical importance of high intakes of whole, fresh fruits and vegetables in the diet. Flavonoids protect people who eat plant-based diets and lower their risk of developing brain diseases.

Homocysteine

Many people—constantly reminded by advertising—believe that high-protein diets are healthy diets. You might be surprised to learn that America eats far too much animal protein. We're repeatedly reminded of the so-called healthy benefits of drinking three glasses of milk per day and eating an animal-product-based diet. But it's actually unhealthy to eat more protein than your body requires. In fact, excess dietary protein causes serious health conditions such as increased aggression, kidney stones and disease, heart disease, colon cancer, and osteoporosis.

High levels of homocysteine result primarily from the intake of animal proteins, not plant proteins. Animal proteins contain an abundance of the essential amino acid methionine. If you eat a lot of methionine-rich foods, you will form higher levels of the toxic amino acid homocysteine. Homocysteine is formed from methionine. Fish have particularly high levels of methionine. To convert toxic homocysteine back into methionine requires folic acid and B vitamins.

Brain-Dangerous Dairy Products

—Milk increases the uptake of neurotoxic cadmium, mercury, and lead in the brain.

—The milk sugar galactose builds up in the lens of the eye, causing cataracts.

—Dairy products create an increased risk of diabetes. Diabetics have more and more serious nervous system problems, such as dementia.

—The high fat content of dairy products leads to increased intake of neurotoxic environmental chemicals like PCB and dioxin.

—Milk causes a leaky gut, which does not support optimal brain health.

—Milk intake increases heart disease risk, which ultimately impacts brain function.

Some researchers believe that it's elevated homocysteine levels, and not high cholesterol, that actually cause brain strokes. In one study, the risk of stroke in women with the highest levels of homocysteine was two times that in women with the lowest levels and equal to the risk posed by smoking a pack of cigarettes per day. In the United States, stroke is a major cause of nervous system impairment. By eating less animal protein and making sure you have a good dietary supply of the vitamins B6 and B12 and folic acid, you can reduce your risk of strokes. Another study pointed out that the participants with higher folic acid levels demonstrated an improved memory recall for a story compared with those with low blood levels of folic acid. High levels of homocysteine have also been implicated in causing more outbreaks of anger and hostility. Known risk factors for heart disease include hostility and frequent anger expression; however, studies show homocysteine may cause both heart disease and increased hostility

The issue of high-protein diets became even more confusing with the recent media coverage of them as an effective and healthy means to trim your waistline. People on high-protein diets may indeed lose weight, but they compromise their health in the process and usually gain weight back, have severe kidney ailments, and even bad breath as a result.

High-Sugar Processed Foods

People suspected of having problems regulating proper blood sugar levels are commonly given a glucose tolerance test. The test is usually given after the person has fasted overnight or for twelve hours. After fasting, blood glucose level is normally around 70 to 110 milligrams per one-tenth of a liter of blood. For simplicity, let's say the level is 100 milligrams. That would equal about 1 gram of sugar per liter of blood. People typically have a blood volume of about 5 liters, meaning that during fasting, a total of only 5 grams of sugar circulates in the blood. On the other hand, a typical consumer may ingest a high-sugar food or drink that contains two times, or even ten times, the normal 5-gram level of sugar. This excess sugar rapidly floods into the bloodstream.

When blood sugar increases in the brain region called the hypothalamus, it signals the pancreas to release insulin. Insulin, in turn, directs removal of sugar from the blood into body cells—except the brain cells. Therefore, insulin release causes a dramatic drop in blood glucose levels. Since the brain heavily relies on glucose as an energy source, this drop in blood sugar can cause a brain energy crisis. Ironically, an even lower blood sugar level results following a quick sugar fix. About two hours after a large intake of sugar, you feel sleepy and irritable because of the lack of blood sugar. Insulin also has another undesirable trait—it encourages the manufacture of sugar into fat tissue.

In addition, high blood sugar causes a dangerous condition in which amino acids combine with the elevated sugars to produce cross-linked, sugar-damaged proteins called advanced glycosylated cross-link end products, or AGEs. The AGE-proteins, if used to make tissue proteins, can cause significant havoc in the tiny blood capillaries of the brain and the myelin covering that electrically insulates the nerve cell. The greater the degree of cross-linking that these proteins possess, the less elasticity the tissues will have. In the blood system, the sugar cross-linked proteins lead to decreased blood vessel flexibility and result in an increase in a specific type of blood pressure called pulse pressure.

Pulse pressure is the pressure difference between the high (systolic) and low (diastolic) blood pressure numbers. An increased pulse pressure increases heart disease risk since it increases the heart's work. Additionally, it also increases the risk of strokes to the brain. People with blood pressures in the high part of the normal range have increased risks of stroke and heart attack.

Diabetics who cannot control their blood sugar have increased risk of mental decline and dementia as they age. Excess sugar has toxic effects upon the vascular system such as clogged and inflexible arteries, which can lead to increased strokes and mental decline. Further, people with both high blood pressure and diabetes have double the risk of cognitive impairment as they age.

About one-third of Americans have a condition called reactive hypoglycemia, which causes them to react to a high intake of simple sugars by releasing excessive amounts of insulin. Of course, the high levels of insulin cause the blood sugar levels to plummet, and the adrenal glands release a burst of epinephrine (adrenaline) in a response effort to establish a higher blood sugar level. It's not surprising that at this point these people feel overstressed and nervous or experience excessive perspiration. Remember, brain functions remain tethered to glucose as their energy source, and the brain has very little capacity to burn fats for energy. Evidence shows that in brain disease, patients lose the ability to maintain proper blood glucose levels either by excessive insulin secretion, as in Alzheimer's disease, or by impaired glucose utilization, as in Parkinson's and Huntington's diseases. Some studies even show that people with normal blood sugar responses rarely have the classic conditions of Alzheimer's dementia. Alzheimer's sufferers, in particular, show most damage in the hippocampus, an area of the brain especially vulnerable to low glucose and oxygen levels.

A diet consisting mainly of processed foods and animal products (contaminated with pollutants) likely plays a central role in many cases of brain disorders. The choice of proper foods and decreasing your exposure to known neurotoxic agents in early life can protect your mental functioning later in life. Proper nutrition not only supports brain health, but preserves brain function as well. As the general population ages, the number of people tormented with brain diseases will rise. But you can take positive steps today to decrease your risk of brain disorders.

4

Stress

The Unsuspected Environmental Toxic Agent

DO UNEXPECTED NOISES startle you in the night? Do memories of frustrating daily episodes keep you awake? Such stresses can take a toll on your brain, particularly on the faculties of learning and memory. As scientists better understand the effects of stress on the brain, a scary picture emerges. Continued exposure to stress overburdens the brain with the prolonged presence of powerful hormones originally designed for short-term emergency situations. Long-term stress actually damages and destroys brain cells and can impair the growth of new brain cells needed for learning and can inhibit memory formation and retrieval.

The Stress Response

Human stress responses evolved through time periods and environmental conditions distinctly different from the physical, psychological, and social world of today. The fight-or-flight response guarded people against life-threatening incidents, such as an attacking tribe or predators. In today's society, we now experience stressful situations that our brains sense as life-threatening even when they are not. Dreading an upcoming deadline does not require an intense physical activity like running or climbing a tree, but we ready ourselves for one anyway. Anticipating a stressful workday can release stress hormones. In current times, instead of being chased up a tree by a toothy predator, we're stuck in traffic jams or face work deadlines that push our systems into panic mode. Whether the danger is imaginary, remembered, or real, your brain reacts swiftly with powerful hormones that set dramatic metabolic changes in motion.

O

The Fight-or-Flight Response

When faced with real or imagined danger, your body reacts quickly:

- —Your heart pumps faster to deliver more blood to the muscles
- —Your breathing rate increases to bring more oxygen to the blood
- —Your senses of smell and hearing become keener
- —Your system releases sugars and fats for quick energy
- —Your muscles becomes tense in anticipation of action
- —Your digestion of food is interrupted to divert more blood to the muscles and brain
- —Your palms become sweaty from perspiration, which lowers the body temperature

Under life-threatening situations when your body must prepare for battle, these responses would be appropriate. Modern-day stresses, however, result from being trapped in a delayed airplane or worrying about a looming work deadline at your desk, and you're left stewing in your own battle juices.

The brain's limbic system, often called the emotional brain, since it controls memory and emotions, responds to stress first. Whenever you experience real danger—or even an imagined threat—your limbic system alerts the autonomic nervous system, the complex array of glands that regulates basic metabolism. The autonomic nervous system has two components, each acting to balance the other.

The first component, the sympathetic nervous system (SNS), activates the fight-or-flight response. In contrast, the second component, the parasympathetic nervous system (PNS), stimulates the relaxation response. Like two ballroom dancers, these two components of the autonomic nervous system maintain a delicate equilibrium. When something disturbs this sensitive balance, the SNS and PNS work to restore the equilibrium of stress hormones. Some stress hormones exert their effects longer than needed to respond to situations encountered in modern life and remain active in the brain for a lengthy period. Their residual effects can lead to brain cell death in the hippocampus, an area of your brain that plays a central role in learning and memory.

The sympathetic nervous system has an impressive capacity to prepare the body swiftly to confront a danger or threat. SNS hormones set metabolic processes in motion that prepare you to deal with sudden threats. The SNS directs the adrenal glands to release epinephrine (formerly known as adrenaline) and other hormones that increase your breathing rate and heart rate; subsequently, blood pressure rises.

These metabolic changes result in more oxygen-rich blood being transported to the brain and to muscles that are used for fighting or fleeing. Epinephrine also directs a rapid release of fats and glucose into your bloodstream. Epinephrine gives you a keener sense of smell and hearing, and more tolerance to pain. At the same time, other hormones arrest functions deemed unnecessary during the sudden danger. For example, the immune, digestion, and reproductive systems are put on standby. Limited blood circulation occurs to areas of the skin. As a result, long-term stress can eventually lead to increased sickness, sexual problems, and skin conditions.

A Delicate Balance

Once your stress response has been activated, it wisely maintains you in a state of readiness—that toothy predator may still lurk in the shadows. Because of the dominance of the SNS over the PNS, it often requires a collective conscious effort to relax after a stressful event.

After the threat has passed, you try to calm down and return to normal. Unfortunately, many people have difficulty returning to a calm state, and it becomes even more difficult with advancing age. Our especially hectic lifestyles may trigger the SNS again and again with increasing frequency. Although the more dominant SNS jumps into action swiftly, it shuts down slowly to allow for the more relaxing PNS to calm things down. When the threat finally diminishes, your brain activates a different course of actions that attempt to bring the stimulating and the relaxing systems in your body back into balance or equilibrium. If you have too much stimulation without periods of relaxation, you will experience the condition known as stress. Long-term stress can have serious implications for the health of the brain.

Not All Stress Is Bad

Keep in mind that a working stress response is healthy. The stress response releases norepinephrine, one of the main excitatory brain messengers. To form new memories you require norepinephrine, and it also elevates your mood. Therefore, life's problems handled productively can feel more like challenges, stimulating creative thinking and encouraging your brain to grow new nerve cell connections and branches within itself.

Researchers have found that some kinds of stress can benefit people. Stresses originating from performing memory tasks will enhance the immune system, but stress generated by passively watching violent videos will weaken the immune system.

Therefore, positive stress management—not total elimination of stress—helps keep a brain healthy.

Fight-or-Flight Versus Tend-and-Befriend

Men and women have a very basic behavioral difference in how they react to stress. Researchers have shown that men often respond to stress with the fight-or-flight response. Someone who reacts with a fight-or-flight pattern when presented with a stressful event will respond either with aggressive behavior, such as a physical fight or verbal assault, or by withdrawing or fleeing from the stressful incident.

In contrast, women approach their stresses with a tend-and-befriend pattern. Researchers have observed that females respond to stressful situations by defending and nurturing their young (the "tend" response) and further by engaging social interaction and support from a network of other females (the "befriend" response). Befriending includes talking on the phone with close friends or relatives or simply asking for directions when lost.

Natural selection likely shaped the female tend-and-befriend pattern. During hunter-gatherer times, pregnant women or women caring for infants did not have the options of fleeing or fighting during threatening episodes. Therefore, to increase survival odds, females developed cooperative social alliances among other females to better defend and nurture their children during dangerous times.

The female reaction to stress directly contrasts with the male fight-or-flight pattern. However, researchers have long considered the fight-or-flight response the primary method used by both sexes to deal with stressful encounters. This oversight occurred because stress-related research historically focused only on men. Not until recently did research explore women's response to stress.

Fathers and mothers also display a different "tending response" with their children following a stressful workday. Research has shown that when the average father returned from a stressful day at the office, he reacted by separating himself from his family. Instead of social contact, the father would try to detach from the family and stay locked up in his study. A father subjected to intense work-related stress will often angrily lash out and clash with his children or wife at home. In contrast, the average mother returning home from a stressful day at work responded by nurturing her children.

These different responses to stress may explain why men succumb more to the harmful health effects of long-term stress. Men more commonly display stress-related conditions such as aggressive behavior, hypertension, or substance abuse. The tend-and-befriend pattern may insulate women against some harmful effects of stress and may underlie the reason women generally live about five to seven years longer than men.

The Hippocampus, Stress, and Memory Retrieval

Researchers have shown that long-term stress can degrade the hippocampus, the portion of the limbic brain vital to memory and learning. (The hippocampus gets its name from the Greek word for sea horse, since its unique shape resembles this creature.) The offenders in this case are the glucocorticoids, a class of hormones released from the adrenal glands during stressful events. Glucocorticoids are more commonly referred to as corticosteroids, or simply as cortisol. During an episode of stress, the adrenal glands swiftly release epinephrine. If the stressful episode is severe or prolonged beyond a few minutes, the adrenal glands will secrete cortisol. Once cortisol gains access to the brain, it stays much longer than epinephrine and is active longer in brain cells. A sustained release of stress hormones can have adverse affects on brain functions, particularly on memory function. Exposure to prolonged and high levels of cortisol can keep the brain from forming new memories or retrieving old memories. Cortisol diverts glucose to other areas of the body like the muscles,

The Hippocampus and Prefrontal Cortex

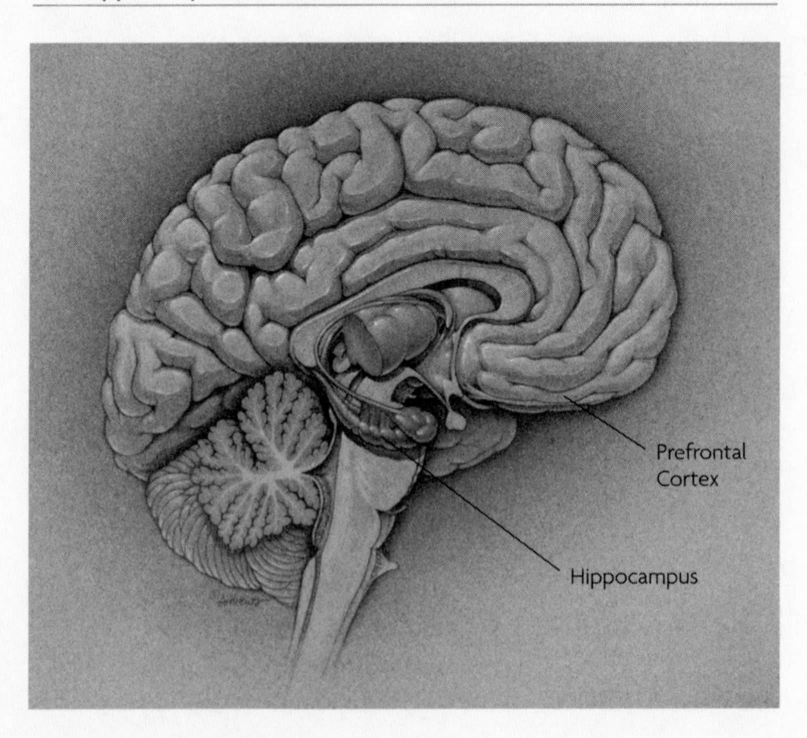

thereby causing a lack of energy in the hippocampus, further reducing the brain's ability to construct new memories.

Low levels of brain glucose may prevent some people from recalling details of an extremely traumatic event that normally would have been remembered. In addition, a glucose-related energy crisis might explain why short-term memory declines first during age-related memory loss. Cortisol also actually inhibits the proper functions of brain messengers used to communicate with different brain cells. High levels of cortisol make it hard to think properly or to recall long-term memories. One reason people become confused during an extreme emergency situation is that their minds go numb from cortisol and they can't respond properly. Their memory is not lost, it's just temporarily inaccessible.

A study used humans to test cortisol's effects on memorizing and recalling sixty words. The test subjects retrieved the words immediately after memorizing them and then again twenty-four hours later. Subjects received either cortisol or a placebo tablet. People treated with cortisol demonstrated impaired memory only when given cortisol an hour before the memory test on the following day. Animal research also confirmed the human studies, revealing that high levels of cortisol impaired memory, but only when subjects tried to retrieve older, long-term rather than recent memories. Cortisol only impaired the memory for a short time. Perhaps high cortisol levels explain why people forget important details during a presentation to a large audience or during courtroom testimony.

Long-Term Stress Damages the Hippocampus

The hippocampus serves as the main junction box that decides whether a new memory will be shuttled into long-term memory or erased after it serves its short-term use. The hippocampus appears to integrate memories together by acting like a central relay station, communicating with required brain sites to form the complete memory. Food-storing birds like chickadees possess a more developed hippocampus and have longer-lasting memories for where they stored their food compared with birds with a smaller hippocampus. London taxi drivers, famous for their abilities to navigate the complex arrangement of city streets, not surprisingly also have enlarged hippocampi.

Persistently high stress levels can injure the brain's hippocampus and make it more difficult to learn new concepts. Researchers have discovered that exposing rats to long-term stress caused them to continuously re-explore their surroundings as if they had no capacity to recall their memory of them. The researchers concluded that the rats behaved similarly to animals that had sustained damage to their hippocampus.

Once the hippocampus loses its ability to control the release of cortisol, it creates a vicious cycle that damages the brain and, ultimately, the quality of life. Researchers have shown that very stressful events or prolonged exposure to cortisol enhances the decline of the aging hippocampus. Since the hippocampus controls signals to halt cortisol release, a compromised hippocampus allows unrestrained cortisol release. This state of uncontrolled cortisol release further degenerates memory and cognitive function.

Typically, in dealing with stressful episodes, the brain's hypothalamus produces a corticotropin-releasing hormone that regulates the pituitary gland to secrete another hormone (adrenocorticotrophic hormone), which directs the adrenals to produce cortisol. With significantly elevated blood cortisol, several structures of the brain, particularly the hippocampus, will alert the hypothalamus to stop the cascade of signals leading to cortisol release.

This process normally controls cortisol levels properly. But the hippocampus sustains the most injury from exposure to high levels of cortisol. Researchers have described how people can lose 20 to 25 percent of the brain cells contained in the hippocampus with aging. In these cases the hippocampus may lose the ability to properly regulate the hypothalamus and to control cortisol secretion. In this context, a damaged hippocampus leads to even more cortisol release and further degeneration of the hippocampus. Increasingly higher levels of cortisol make it ever more difficult to activate the relaxation response.

In a group of seventy-year-olds, those who had the highest levels of cortisol also had a smaller hippocampus. This group also performed worse on two tasks that use the hippocampus—memorizing a route through a human maze and recalling pictures viewed a day earlier.

Researchers using magnetic resonance imaging demonstrated that particular alterations in the hippocampus came with aging, behavioral changes, and Alzheimer's disease. If specific components of the hippocampus shrink or degenerate, you lose discrete memory skills. Moreover, people with a reduced or smaller hippocampus will likely progress toward Alzheimer's more rapidly. The brain's capacity to rewire its circuitry and to repair itself after damage directly relates to its ability to form new memories. Therefore, the hippocampus's need to grow new nerve cells may relate directly to its memory functions.

Stress Hormones Suppress the Growth of New Neurons

Stress inhibits nerve cells from sprouting and growing. To form new memories, the brain has to stimulate the growth of new brain cells, a process called neurogenesis. Researchers have demonstrated that thousands of new hippocampal nerve cells form every day in healthy adults. Animal studies on rats showed that nerve cells in the hippocampi doubled after the rats carried out demanding learning tasks. However, behavioral tasks that did not involve the hippocampus did not enhance new nerve cell growth.

Stress hormone levels tend to rise with aging and may cause declines in neurogenesis in older people. However, if you remove sources of high stress and they do not persist for long periods, the brain can recover since it still has the ability to grow new nerve cells.

Persistent Stress Is Hard on Your "Cranial-Radiator"

Proper memory recall and brain health depend on the vast networks of blood vessels dedicated to it. The four hundred miles of brain capillaries alone contribute to an estimated one hundred square feet of surface area. Proper functioning of this complex blood vessel network can lead directly to healthy brain function. The blood vessel network constantly delivers essential nutrients such as amino acids, oxygen, and glucose to the brain. The blood network removes toxic chemicals and also has the less well known function of serving to cool the brain—like a cranial radiator. In order for the human brain to evolve to a greater size, it needed a cooling system to prevent the heat generated by mental activity from overheating the brain. Since the physical act of thought processing generates a lot of heat, an efficient cranial blood heat exchange became necessary for higher levels of brain function.

The BrainGate, Stress, and the Gulf War Syndrome

Stressful episodes produce a host of adaptive changes that prepare us to better survive in a crisis. Yet stress has been shown to decrease the effectiveness of the BrainGate. In several studies, the brains of stressed mice showed greater amounts of elements that usually don't cross the BrainGate.

Stress is likely the cause of the Gulf War syndrome. During the Gulf War, soldiers routinely received an antidote (pyridostigmine) for nerve gas to prevent the potential harmful effects of chemical warfare agents. Battlefield soldiers reported nervous system side effects far more often than soldiers given the same drug outside the theater of combat. As it turns out, the effects of battle stress crippled the BrainGate enough to allow the antidote to enter the brain and cause harm.

It's clear that excess, extended stress can weaken the BrainGate. Stressful episodes can suddenly increase the ability of items to cross through the BrainGate. Prescription and over-the-counter drugs have been designed and tested for safety, assuming that they would not gain access to the brain. Under stressful episodes, however, some of these drugs may very well cross into the brain. Therefore, do not overlook the use of proper stress management to keep a healthy brain and mental state.

Noise: An Insidious Source of Stress

Unexpected loud sounds instantly trigger the stress response. Since sudden and loud sounds usually signal a dangerous situation such as an attacking predator, humans have evolved an effective and rapid response to loud noise stresses. The modern world has become polluted with noise of all types that constantly assaults our sanity. From leaf blowers to diesel trucks, most urban people today cannot avoid noise stress.

Human newborns react quickly to sound and respond to every different sound they detect. However, sudden loud noises usually trigger a startle response in babies. Startled babies show emotional excitement, tighten their muscles, and change body positions; their heart rates increase. The startle response occurs even in a fetus in the mother's womb. Since it equips us to go from a deep sleep into battle-ready mode in seconds, the startle response clearly has helped in our survival. However, people living in modern mega-cities find it impossible to avoid being assaulted with relentless and unpleasant noises.

Noise Affects the Prefrontal Cortex

Noise can worsen some psychiatric illnesses, particularly disorders linked to an area of the brain called the prefrontal cortex (PFC). The last area of the brain to evolve in humans, the prefrontal cortex shows damage first from the effects of pollution and stress. Researchers investigating effects of noise stress on brain function in monkeys demonstrated that noise stress impairs the cognitive functioning of the PFC. Furthermore, they showed that noise stress exerted these changes on a key brain messenger, dopamine. Dopamine plays a central role in many brain disorders such as Parkinson's disease and attention-deficit/hyperactivity disorder.

Usually noise threats signal an urgent reason to respond, first with the unconscious mind rather than the conscious mind. Researchers speculate that the conscious mind may not react swiftly enough to properly manage life or death incidents. Using magnetic resonance brain-imaging techniques, scientists have studied noise response in test subjects stressed with sudden loud noises in combination with graphic images. The body will automatically respond to the noise stress—you have no choice but to react. Interestingly, women react more easily to noise stress and perceive noise as being stressful sooner than men. Women are also more easily frightened by loud noises that only startled men.

Persistent Noise Is Persistent Stress

Loud and frightening noises are not alone in activating the stress response. Persistent low-level noise also has deleterious effects on stress behavior. Low-intensity noise from traffic or from office equipment, for example, contributes to stress as well. Noisy environments at home or school can adversely affect a child's ability to learn. When compared with children from quieter environs, those children living near heavily traveled freeways or near airports show a tendency to develop language and reading skills more slowly.

More hospital admissions for psychiatric disturbances occur in noisy communities. Fatigue, angry moods, aggression, and inability to concentrate, not to mention lowered work performance, may result from persistent exposure to low-level noise.

Traffic Noise. Typical everyday traffic noise can have serious mental health effects. A study that investigated the non–hearing-loss health consequences of low-level community noise found that exposed children had elevated stress hormones coupled with increases in blood pressure and heart rate. Even low-ambient traffic noise typically found in most cities and neighborhoods can provoke stress by triggering nervousness and anxiety. Children who lived in noisier environs displayed elevated nighttime levels of the stress hormone cortisol, slightly higher blood pressure, and a greater heart rate increase in response to a stress test. These children showed signs of elevated stress compared with those from quieter neighborhoods. Therefore, as the studies show, the ambient background noise can significantly increase the levels of stress. Exposure of children to persistent traffic or ambient noise should be a concern, since it has also been shown to decrease learning and motivation.

Office Noise. Low-level ambient noise at work has been found to decrease productivity and task motivation in workers. Employees assigned to quiet offices or those with low-intensity office noise (including speech) produced fewer stress hormones compared with workers in noisy offices. The stress from a noisy office clearly led to more stress-related behaviors and had adverse effects on employee motivation. Typical low-level office noise may cause persistent stress, which we know can lead to significant health problems, decreasing worker productivity even further.

An expanding body of evidence indicates the vital role stress plays in declining mental health. Therefore, using effective techniques for managing stress and enhancing your relaxation response can increase your brain wellness.

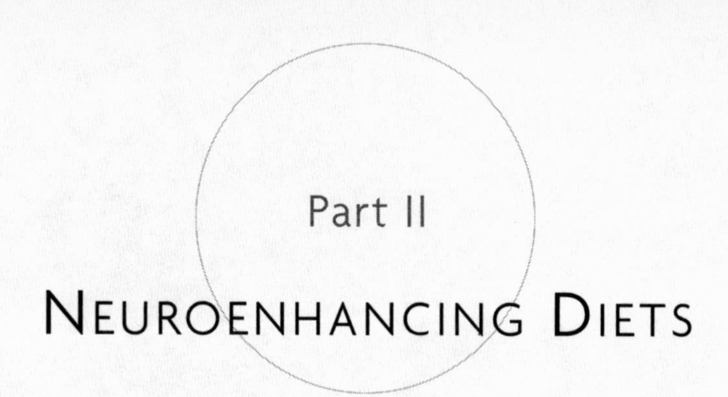

Part II

Neuroenhancing Diets

5

A Feast for the Mind

THE ADULT BRAIN is a hungry organ requiring items it cannot make such as oxygen and glucose. Therefore, understanding essential brain nutrition helps you understand how to optimize your brain's functioning.

About 70 percent of the total number of brain cells that will become a developed brain have already divided before birth. The most vigorous period of cell division in the brain occurs in the first few weeks of embryonic development, almost before a woman knows she is pregnant. At this point, the embryo receives its nutrition entirely from the mother. Since many toxic metals like lead are stored for decades in the bones, foods the mother ate decades ago can harm the growing fetus. Maternal nutrition, therefore, even prior to conception, can affect the infant.

People consider memory decline normal in older people. People often overlook the fact that healthy diets also keep a brain sharp with advancing age. Studies show that older people who eat brain-healthy diets exhibit less age-related memory losses.

A diet including a healthy balance of nutrients with small amounts of cholesterol, trans-fats, and saturated fats caused less cognitive decline in people seventy and older. A low intake of alcoholic beverages seemed to improve cognitive functioning. While more studies need to clarify the relationship between diet and mental functioning, evidence indicates that light to moderate drinking decreases strokes, increases general health, and may give a boost to some mental capacities.

Fresh fruits and vegetables help to maintain mental abilities since they are rich sources of antioxidants such as vitamins E and C. These antioxidants block the action of toxic free radicals and have been shown to protect against cancers and heart disease and to improve chronic disorders such as Alzheimer's disease. Evidence suggests that omega-3 fats found in walnuts may also prevent mental decline.

One must keep in mind the many underlying causes of mental decline. One often overlooked form of cognitive decline is the blood vessel-related type known as vascular dementia. A healthy blood vessel system protects optimal brain function since vascular disease causes small strokes that directly impact brain function and blood flow to the brain. Vascular disease is estimated to cause 10 to 20 percent of dementia. Don't forget that an optimal diet can significantly protect from vascular dementia. Some dietary agents that have shown preventive promise by increasing cognitive functions include antioxidant vitamins C and E, B-family vitamins, soy isoflavones, monounsaturated fats like olive oil, and omega-3 fats like DHA. Intake of olive oil also protects against age-related cognitive decline. Ginkgo biloba has been shown to improve memory and cognitive function in several studies.

Top Neuroenhancing Foods

—Antioxidants from blueberries, vitamins C and E

—Essential fats from walnuts, flaxseed, and soybeans

—Complex carbohydrates from whole foods (provide sustained sources of energy)

—Cold-pressed olive oil for monounsaturated oil and vitamin E

—Organic fruits and vegetables (antioxidant plant chemicals, pollutant-removing plant fiber; contains fewer brain-toxic pesticides)

—Nutritional supplements: docosahexanoic acid (DHA); coenzyme Q10, phosphatidylserine (PS), *S*-Adenosylmethionine (SAM), and acetyl-L-carnitine (ALC)

—B-family vitamins (B6, B12, folic acid)

—Filtered, purified water

DHA, PS, and Other Fats

The type of dietary fat one consumes plays a vital role in memory decline and other conditions such as learning disorders. Research suggests that the specific type of dietary fat may influence children's moods and abilities to learn. Many parents have started to believe the old adage "you are what you eat." Many parents reluctantly choose to give their child Ritalin, the drug used to treat learning disorders. Alternatively, some families use an entirely different strategy: they monitor the child's diet, especially the essential fat intake.

The typical American diet provides a poor source of the two essential fats—notably omega-3 (DHA or EPA). A number of experts believe that omega-3 fats furnish required dietary components for physical as well as mental health in adults and children. For many families stuck in the habit of eating processed foods, dietary supplements may provide the only means to satisfy their requirements for the essential fats. It's not surprising that some children, within weeks of including essential fats in their diet, performed better in school. These children turned into more outgoing and more self-assured students and participated more in class. A number of studies have revealed that older adults given essential fats also displayed dramatic mental improvements.

Essential Fats

Humans make all of the fats they require for nutrition except two: omega-6 fats and omega-3 fats. Because these vital fats require dietary sources, they have been called essential fats. The typical American processed-food diet favors more of the omega-6 rather than omega-3 fats. Therefore, most people in the United States consume far too much of the omega-6 fats. Plant nuts and seeds provide the best sources of essential fats. Essential fats play a key role in brain development and health, and nervous tissue such as the myelin sheath and the brain's gray and white matter contain them in abundance.

Fish oils contain the omega-3 fats called eicosapentaenoic acid, or EPA, and docosahexanoic acid, or DHA. DHA and EPA support both brain and immune functions. Fish especially high in DHA and EPA include salmon, herring, mackerel, sablefish, sardines, and tuna. However, because of the potential for some of these fish to harbor neurotoxic pollutants such as mercury and PCB, it is better to use DHA supplements to increase your intake (see Part III—Neuromins [DHA]).

The vital essential fats form the primary foundations during brain development and play pivotal roles in brain development since the nervous tissue abundantly contains them in the gray and white matter of the brain. The brain contains mostly fat, which accounts for about 60 percent of its dry weight. Essential fats provide one of the very basic building blocks of nerve cells and form structural foundations for the protective blood-brain barrier that we call the BrainGate. In addition to the structural support fats provide, they also play critical roles in the communication that occurs within the brain.

Sources of Essential Fats

Omega-3 Fats	Omega-6 Fats
Flax seeds (linseed)	Flax seeds (linseed)
Walnuts	Walnuts
Soybeans and soy products	Soybeans and soy products
Wheat germ oil	Cottonseed and peanut oil
DHA (Neuromins supplement)	Sunflower seed oil
Whole grains	Corn and safflower oil

Eating too much of the omega-6 fats has a downside, since they encourage inflammation. The omega-6 fats are converted into highly reactive compounds that promote inflammation. Thus a diet very high in omega-6 fats can favor inflammation and make it easy for the blood to clot, increasing the risk of heart disease. On the other hand, omega-3 fats assist in keeping the inflammatory reaction in balance and support brain nutrition. The World Health Organization suggests a 5:1 or 10:1 omega-6 to omega-3 ratio in the diet.

DHA, probably the most important brain fat, is the primary structural fat in the gray matter that supports communication between nerve cells. Study subjects who received DHA showed increased intelligence. Recent studies have displayed that the meager quantity of omega-3 fats in infant formulas has been linked to lower intelligence in formula-fed children.

Breast-Feeding Equals Brain-Feeding

Breast milk is a very rich source of DHA for developing babies. A study in Italy compared feeding either DHA-rich breast milk or formulas deficient in DHA to four-month-old infants. They found a significant difference in infant brain development in infants fed breast milk compared with infants fed DHA-deficient formula group. The breast-fed infants scored much higher on a scale that measures psychomotor development. Studies show that DHA assists the developing brain, so the status of a baby's essential fats depends on the mother's nutrition. DHA levels increase in babies who feed from mothers who have a diet high in omega-3 fats.

As it turns out, a constant supply of DHA is required not only during the fetal period but also throughout childhood and adulthood. Animals born from parents maintained on an omega-3–deficient diet for the last two weeks of pregnancy showed over a 30 percent decrease in brain size. Other studies have indicated that low levels of DHA in the brain slowed and altered learning patterns. Brain disorders occur more often in low-birth-weight babies. Low-birth-weight babies usually come from malnourished mothers who have essential fat deficiencies. Studies have revealed that infant rhesus monkeys receiving a diet poor in omega-3 fats suffered from visual impairments. Human infants also displayed visual impairment when they received formula excessively rich in only omega-6 fats compared with infants fed omega-3–rich breast milk. Some of the neurodevelopmental disorders linked to low intake of essential fats include poor cognitive ability, mental retardation, cerebral palsy, and autism.

DHA also assists in the uptake and use of glucose, and has a role in the signaling activity between nerves. Adequate DHA levels may also prevent

Benefits of Breast-Feeding

—Breast-fed babies have higher IQs and better vision than those fed formula.

—Breast-fed infants are mentally enhanced (the longer the infants were breast-fed, the greater the mental enhancement).

—Breast-fed babies have larger heads! Low levels of essential fats measured at birth are related to smaller head circumferences and low birth weights.

—Babies given only breast milk for the first two months of life are much less prone to developing non–insulin-dependent diabetes.

—Breast milk provides essential fats for brain growth.

—Breast milk is rich in brain-friendly DHA.

—Breast milk provides essential minerals and vitamins.

—Breast milk transfers the mother's protective antibodies to the infant.

diseases associated with impaired glucose regulation, such as some types of diabetes, obesity, and hypertension. Individuals with these diseases usually exhibit a greater decline in mental functions as they age. Breast milk is rich in DHA and babies given only breast milk for the first two months of life have a dramatically lower incidence of non–insulin-dependent diabetes.

Both adults and children need DHA and AA (arachidonic acid) for brain growth and maintenance. These substances are included in some infant formulas. For example, infants given both DHA and AA showed significantly improved problem-solving abilities. Another study showed that an insufficient amount of the essential fats measured at birth relates to smaller head circumferences and low birth weights.

Other studies showed that supplementing with DHA and AA dramatically elevated the average intelligence scores in a group of children. The infants received both DHA and AA, only DHA, or neither DHA nor AA. After seventeen weeks, the Mental Development Index was used to test the infants for language skills, memory, and problem-solving. Not surprisingly, the highest average score came from the group that received both DHA and AA, followed by the DHA-only group. The lowest average mental development scores came from the control group, which did not receive DHA or AA.

A general trend, supported by over twenty studies, indicates that breast-fed babies have a higher IQ and better vision then those fed infant formulas. The increased intelligence showed up in infants as young as six months and persisted through fifteen years of age. The longer the infants received breast milk, the greater the mental enhancement.

What type of diet will give a child the best chance for healthy brain growth and development? For newborn babies, breast milk provides the most critical food for brain development. Research has shown that breast milk supplies far superior nutrition compared with formulas for an infant's brain development.

A decline in brain DHA levels causes a loss of the functional and structural integrity of the cell membranes. Free radicals can oxidize and break down DHA, which results in its decline. Many patients with brain disorders such as senile dementia, Parkinson's, and Alzheimer's demonstrate a loss of fats such as DHA.

Low levels of DHA appear with select neurological conditions. Low levels of DHA are significant risk factors for senile dementia and Alzheimer's. There is also an association between low levels of DHA and increased hostility and aggression.

The research identifies a critical problem—people cannot make sufficient DHA in advancing age. Therefore, supplements of DHA may forestall some conditions such as Alzheimer's and heart disease. Thus, DHA is a vital dietary component for people of all ages.

Further studies show that diets high in omega-6 fats (high in red meat) cause mental decline in older men (sixty-nine to eighty-nine years old).

Processed Oils

The centuries-old, time-honored method used stone presses to crush seeds and nuts to extract and refine their oils. However, to increase oil yields, modern commercial food processors extract oils by subjecting the seeds to a combination of crushing, high temperatures, and high pressures. Often the commercial oils become further degraded from exposure to light and oxygen. In order to increase the oil yield even further, some food processors add a chemical solvent (typically hexane, a known neurotoxic agent) to the crushed-seed pulp to enhance the extraction of more oil. By boiling the oil, processors can remove the volatile solvents (which destroys vitamin E), yet solvent residues remain and solvent treatment transfers more pesticides into the extracted oil. The high-temperature treatment of oils also causes some of the fatty acids to oxidize and break down into toxic forms.

High-temperature cooking and frying in oil also produce toxic compounds called acrylamides. Some common widely consumed foods such as bread, French fries, biscuits, and potato chips contain high levels of acrylamide, a substance that is toxic to both the central nervous system and the peripheral nervous system. Studies have revealed that a typical bag of potato chips can contain up to 500 times more acrylamide than the highest amount allowed in drinking water, according to the World Health Organization. Foods cooked at very high temperatures such as oven-baked, fried, or deep-fried potatoes and overprocessed cereal foods contain the highest levels of acrylamide.

The healthy technique of cold-pressing or expeller-pressing oils isolates the seed oil without destroying the vitamin E content and oxidizing the oils. Extra-virgin olive oil produced by slowly pressing the olives (sometimes cold-pressed) between stone or steel rollers preserves the oil and vitamin E. Olive oil also supports myelin, a fatty outer layer that insulates nerves and contains mostly fat. Oleic acid is the most plentiful fat in the myelin layer. As it turns out, olive oil contains mostly monounsaturated oleic acid. Oleic acid is also present in avocados, almonds, macadamias, peanuts, and pecans.

Partially Hydrogenated Oils: Bad News for the Brain

To further increase profits, commercial food processors chemically transform oils normally liquid at room temperature into thicker or saturated solid fats at room temperature. For example, after hydrogenation, corn oil turns into solid margarine at room temperature. To accomplish this, corn oil is subjected to high temperatures and high pressures, and infused with hydrogen gas using metal catalysts (nickel) that speed up the hydrogenation reaction. Under these conditions, hydrogen added to the corn oil transforms it into a solid at room temperature. The resulting margarine is then steam-cleaned at high temperatures to remove odors and bleached to mask its unappealing gray color. Finally, a yellow dye is added to the margarine to give it the appearance of butter. In the early 1900s, thirty-two states banned precolored margarine. Margarine was shipped with capsules of yellow dye that had to be mixed by the consumer. The ban was lifted in the 1950s. Ironically, butter makers now add yellow dyes to compete with the rich yellow artificial color of margarine!

Food processors benefit greatly from hydrogenated oils since they have creamy textures (flaky pie crusts result from hydrogenated oils) and much longer shelf lives. The health effects to consumers of these oils, however, are enormous. Hydrogenated and partially hydrogenated oils create a toxic type of trans-fat, rarely found in higher animals, or nature for that matter (although some bacteria produce it). Many of the artificial trans-fats are incorporated into the cell membranes, substituting for the normal fats. Trans-fats clearly harm human health and brain function.

Trans-Fats Versus Cis-Fats. The cell membranes of the brain, normally pliable, require their fluid-like properties in order to function. The cells normally gain this flexibility from the physical makeup of different fats residing in their cell membranes. Thus the physical dimensions and actual shapes of the membrane fats directly influence the membranes' flexibility and fluidity.

Trans-fats have their hydrogen atoms located on the opposite side of the fat molecule. The human body normally uses cis-fat molecules that have the hydrogen atoms on the same side. The normal cis-fat form of linoleic acid, for example, is more than three times wider than the trans-fat form of linoleic acid. For this reason, many researchers have speculated that BrainGate membranes composed of the thinner trans-fats will leak more items than membranes composed of normal cis-fats. If true, this could have dramatic effects on the health and function of the brain, allowing many toxic items to cross into the brain. Perhaps one could also speculate that a lifetime of eating BrainGate-weakening trans-fats fosters increased aluminum uptake into the brains of older individuals.

Research has demonstrated that these unnatural trans-fats do indeed cross the BrainGate and brain cells use them. Trans-fats, when incorporated into your cell membranes, will likely increase the permeability of the barrier and allow molecules and viruses access to the cell. Trans-fats change the very makeup of the membrane and likely alter the brain-messenger receptors that reside on the surface of the brain cell (neuron). This alteration can disrupt the chemical communication of the brain messengers that interact with the receptors. Trans-fats lay down a dysfunctional cellular foundation that can disrupt cellular communication and therefore promote a decline in cognitive function. Trans-fats will incorporate themselves into the myelin covering of nerves and brain cells. The presence of trans-fats also changes the electrical properties and conductivity of nerve cells.

The chemical modification of our dietary fatty acids has compromised important structural components in the brain. Trans-fats cause havoc in the circulatory system, and a properly functioning circulatory system is necessary for optimal cognitive function. Trans-fats have been found to block the ability of blood vessels to expand or dilate, increasing the risks for heart disease. Trans-fats lower high-density lipoproteins (HDLs, the good cholesterol) and increase the low-density lipoproteins (LDLs, the bad cholesterol). Other studies have shown that older men who had the highest intake of trans-fats had twice the risk of contracting heart disease. Trans-fats also lead to increased cancer rates. People already deficient in omega-3 fats will absorb twice as many trans-fats when they eat them! Finally, trans-fats may also cause an almost 40 percent increased risk of type 2 diabetes in women who increased their calories from trans-fats by only 2 percent.

The brain's cell membranes can maintain the proper fat balance, provided the diet contains both of the essential fats (omega-3 and omega-6). However, if your diet consists of hydrogenated oils and fats or oils subjected to high-temperature cooking (such as frying), you'll be feeding your brain toxic trans-fats and oxidized fats. So stay away from—or at least limit your intake of—almost all margarines and vegetable shortenings; many crackers, cookies, and snack foods; prepared salad dressings; French fries; doughnuts and other similar fried foods.

Phosphatidylserine

Phosphatidylserine (PS) is a naturally occurring brain fat. Phosphatidylserine and phosphatidylcholine are critical parts of brain cell membranes, including the neurons. Phosphatidylcholine is converted into acetylcholine, a brain messenger. Studies have shown that lowered levels of acetylcholine can lead to memory decline in cases of Alzheimer's. Studies also suggest that PS slightly enhances cognition in people without Alzheimer's.

PS has been shown to treat memory loss in Alzheimer's disease. Studies confirm that Alzheimer's patients given PS supplements showed improved memory and cognitive functioning such as learning. PS enhances the brain's ability to use glucose and works with DHA to increase communication between cells in the brain. PS also increases brain messengers that send cues to other cells vital to memory and to preventing age-related memory impairment. PS builds proper fluidity in brain cell membranes and assists in the transport of nutrients such as glucose into and out of nerve cells. Both PS and phosphatidylcholine are available as supplements. Purchase the Leci-PS version, which is derived from soy. Clinical studies have shown benefits to cognitive function with Leci-PS supplementation (see Appendix).

Other Fats

Saturated fats are exactly that—saturated with hydrogen—and have no room for additional hydrogen. Saturated fats are solid at room temperature and cause high cholesterol and heart disease. Examples include coconut oil, butter, lard, or animal fats.

Polyunsaturated fats have two or more open hydrogen spots and always remain liquid, even if refrigerated. Once thought to have a protective effect against heart disease, polyunsaturated fats now have been found to lower the healthy HDLs. Examples include corn oil, safflower oil, and soybean oil.

Monounsaturated fats have just one unfilled spot for hydrogen to add or make them saturated. They remain liquid at room temperature, but turn into a solid when refrigerated. Monounsaturated fats elevate the levels of HDL in the bloodstream that act like cholesterol sweepers, while lowering LDLs that act like cholesterol litterbugs. The best example of a monounsaturated fat is olive oil. Canola oil is also a monounsaturated fat, but it is overprocessed and therefore not recommended.

Monounsaturated fats such as olive oil may prevent cognitive declines that occur with advancing age. In Italy, senior citizens given extra-virgin olive oil as the primary dietary source of fat demonstrated less age-related cognitive decline than people in the group that consumed less olive oil or monounsaturated oils.

In a recent study, researchers concluded, "It appears that high monounsaturated fatty acid intakes, mostly present in vegetable oils and particularly in extra-virgin olive oil, the main fat of the Mediterranean diet, protect from age-related cognitive decline."

Therefore, changing your diet to include cold-pressed olive oil now might prevent your loss of memory and cognitive skills later in life. Numerous foods, including olives, sesame seeds, avocados, peanuts, almonds, pecans, palm, corn, sunflower seeds, soybeans, cottonseed, and walnuts contain monounsaturated oils.

SAM, ALC, and Coenzyme Q10

S-Adenosylmethionine (SAM) detoxifies cell membranes and assists in making brain messengers such as serotonin. SAM also helps to make phospholipids for cell membranes in the brain. Studies show that SAM-supplemented rats produce more acetylcholine receptors in the memory-intensive hippocampus. SAM also has a positive influence on the mood-elevating brain messengers serotonin and norepinephrine, which may explain its antidepressant use.

SAM also contributes to the manufacture of making melatonin, proteins, glutathione, and various cartilage components. Required in more than forty biochemical reactions, SAM is available as a supplement. In Europe, SAM has been used successfully to improve mood, cognitive function, and general nerve health for over three decades.

Acetyl-L-carnitine, or ALC, an amino acid, shows antiaging effects in the brain. ALC potentially preserves memory in older individuals and assists in slowing memory decline. ALC has been given to

Alzheimer's patients in studies, and the ALC-supplemented group showed a slower mental decline than the group who did not receive ALC. In another study, ALC was given to Alzheimer's patients for three months. The ALC-supplemented group indeed performed better on a series of mental tasks. This finding led investigators to suggest that ALC may slow the progression of senile dementia, particularly in those with mild cases. Like SAM, ALC can be purchased as a supplement at most health food stores.

The antioxidant coenzyme Q10 plays a critical role in energy production. A rare antioxidant, coenzyme Q10 actually protects the mitochondria or the cellular furnace that forms energy. Researchers have found that Parkinson's patients have reduced levels of coenzyme Q10 in their mitochondria. A recent study showed that Parkinson's sufferers given a large dose (1,200 milligrams) of coenzyme Q10 had a slower progression of motor disabilities associated with Parkinson's disease.

Coenzyme Q10 can be found in natural form in vegetables and oils such as spinach, alfalfa, potatoes, soybeans, rice bran oil, and wheat germ oil. Although expensive, coenzyme Q10 is also available as a supplement.

Antioxidants and Free Radicals

Plants adapted to a hostile life on land millions of years before animals. Because of this evolutionary history, plants can deal with environmental stress better than animals. For example, plants make all of the antioxidant vitamins they need to survive. Animals, on the other hand, have either lost that ability or have always depended on plants as sources of antioxidant vitamins and other essential nutrition. Therefore, it makes the most nutritional sense to consume a plant-based diet. In fact, most people did eat a plant-based diet until the last half-century, when processed foods steadily replaced plant products on grocery shelves. Today, most American grocery stores have relegated the produce section to a small area—only about 15 percent—of the store.

Spices

Antioxidants are critical to brain health. While the most important brain antioxidants have the ability to cross the BrainGate, those that don't still have an important role, since they act synergistically and have a sparing effect on other antioxidants, increasing the total level of antioxidant protection.

Luckily for us, some of the most potent antioxidants are also delicious. Herbs and spices, both dried and fresh, are easy to find in your grocery store or at the farmers' market. Here's a look at some specific properties of just some of these plants.

Cayenne peppers (capsicum) are so hot that a concentrated version is used in commercial pepper spray repellant. At lower doses, cayenne elevates moods, protects against stomach ulcers, decreases platelet aggregation, and, because it has antithrombotic properties, hinders the formation of strokes.

Curcumin is a spice used as a yellow coloring agent. The dried and powdered form known as turmeric, a coloring agent in curry, is a spice, food colorant, and food preservative. Aside from turmeric's antioxidant properties, it also has anti-inflammatory action.

Curry powder is also a potent antioxidant and helps to control inflammation. In experimental studies curry was able to decrease the buildup of dangerous amyloid-beta plaques in rodent brains. In rats, curry prevented plaque formation in the synapses that interconnect nerve cells and play a central role in memory. Loss of synapse function may cause cognitive decline in Alzheimer's. Curcumin-supplemented rats also showed better cognitive skills in

Antioxidant Herbs and Spices

Allspice	Cumin	Parsley
Basil	Fennel	Rosemary
Bay leaf	Ginger	Sage
Cilantro	Marjoram	Thyme
Cinnamon	Nutmeg	Turmeric
Clove	Oregano	

memory-related maze testing than groups that did not receive curcumin.

Ginger root is widely used as a spice and has a sweet taste and aroma. It's known to contain some very potent antioxidant compounds. Many ginger compounds have shown more potent antioxidant properties than even vitamin E. Ginger also inhibits platelet clumping, cutting down on blood clots.

Licorice root also has a number of health benefits. It contains antioxidants and helps control inflammation. Licorice can protect against chemical toxicity and inhibits a specific enzyme, ornithine decarboxylase, which may play a role in the prevention of skin, bladder, breast, and prostate cancer. Plant sources of ornithine decarboxylase inhibitors include not only licorice, but carrots, wheat, garlic, onions, asparagus, cucumbers, tomatoes, radishes, potatoes, strawberries, citrus, cruciferous vegetables, and turmeric as well.

Tea

Tea has been grown and cultivated in the Far East for thousands of years. But researchers more recently identified unique compounds in tea called polyphenols that are powerful antioxidants and prevent food from becoming rancid.

Health Benefits of Green Tea Polyphenols

- —Contain potent antioxidants (they're 20 times more potent than vitamin E)
- —Enhance the immune system (support general brain health)
- —Help control platelet clumping (lowering the risk of blood clots)
- —Lower blood pressure
- —Block formation of toxic nitrosamine (linked to brain cancer)

Green and black tea leaves originate form the bushy plant *Camellia sinensis*. Tea leaves are picked and left to dry in hot air. However, black tea is subjected to an oxidation step, which brings out a darker color and unique aroma.

Green tea is processed a bit less. The fresh leaves are steamed to destroy the enzymes that lead to the fermentation in black teas. Since green tea is not allowed to oxidize like black tea, it has a fresh, grassy quality and retains a greater amount of the unique polyphenols.

These unique tea polyphenols provide a number of healthy benefits that cannot be supplied by any other edible plant.

For example, green tea extract has been shown to protect in animal models of Parkinson's disease. Mice were given green tea extracts before a known neurotoxic agent and the extract reduced neuron loss in the substantia nigra, the brain area damaged in Parkinson's.

Flavonoids and Proanthocyanidins

Free radicals are generated at some stage in virtually every case of brain injury or disease. Highly reactive free radicals degrade the myelin sheath and cell membranes in the brain. Therefore, a generous dietary intake of antioxidants provides support for recovery from a brain injury and also prevents future brain injury and mental decline.

Plants have evolved methods to protect themselves from the toxicity of free radicals. For example, the pigments in fruits like blueberries and substances in seeds and nuts are potent antioxidants. Flavonoids include a class of over four thousand naturally occurring plant substances such as polyphenols.

Oxygen is generally assumed necessary for health. But oxygen also reacts easily and triggers substances to become oxidized or rusted, like unprotected metal surfaces. The polyphenols, especially those found in green tea, act as rust-proofing paints, blocking oxygen from causing toxicity. That's why they're called antioxidants.

Flavonoids strengthen capillaries and thus regulate absorption. Flavonoids also work together with vitamin C and help to maintain vitamin C levels from the degrading effects of oxygen. Virtually all fruits and vegetables are excellent sources of flavonoids.

A large body of research shows that age-related memory decline is associated with fat breakdown from oxidation (lipid peroxidation). When sufficient antioxidants are given, the risk of memory decline is lessened. Studies show that antioxidant fruit and vegetable extracts will prevent age-related cognitive decline. One study fed rats extracts of blueberry, spinach, and strawberries for eight weeks. The study result suggest that diets high in antioxidant foods effectively reverse some effects of age-related brain declines. Fresh fruits and vegetables—especially spinach—may play a vital role preventing (and might even reverse) age-related mental declines.

Blueberries contain flavonoids called proanthocyanidins, potent antioxidants named for their blue or cyan colors. Proanthocyanidins have the unique ability to cross the BrainGate and provide antioxidant protection in both the fat and water content of the brain. Proanthocyanidins protect the fat membranes of the myelin sheath and impede free radical activity in the areas inside and outside the brain cell.

Studies show that blueberry proanthocyanidins have greater antioxidant properties than the much-vaunted vitamins E and C. The presence of these plant antioxidants helps the body maintain higher levels of the antioxidant vitamins (such as C and E) and allows the vitamins to participate in their normal metabolic roles rather than neutralizing free radicals. Researchers have determined that fresh blueberries contain some of the highest concentrations of antioxidants—more than garlic, spinach, and blackberries.

Other studies have shown that animals administered blueberry extracts displayed less age-related motor skill decline and performed better on memory tests than animals in the nonsupplemented group. The researchers believe that blueberry extract might even reverse some of the age-related memory loss and motor skill decline.

Grape Seeds, Pine Bark, and Ginkgo. Grapes, especially grape seeds and the dark-purple and red varieties, contain high levels of proanthocyanidins. Ginkgo leaves, pine bark, and grape seeds also contain rich sources. Pycnogenol®, the commercial name for products containing forty distinct antioxidants that originate in the bark of a French pine tree, neutralizes some of the most potent free radicals. In cultured brain cells, Pycnogenol® protected cells from dying after exposure to very toxic chemicals.

Ginkgo biloba, one of the world's oldest trees, contains powerful proanthocyanidins in its leaves that prevent oxidation in blood vessels of the brain. Studies also suggest that ginkgo biloba has the ability to increase cognitive functions. Some European countries routinely administer ginkgo to patients with mental conditions such as depression, memory decline, confusion, anxiety, and difficulty concentrating. However, the efficacy of ginkgo for treating Alzheimer's disease is more uncertain, since not all studies show that patients improve when given ginkgo.

Proteins

Even seemingly healthy people often have some dietary deficiency that influences their behavior and emotions. Since your food can directly influence specific brain-messenger levels, and since these transfer data among more than one trillion brain cells, your diet becomes of paramount importance to a smooth operation. Brain messengers allow you to think, concentrate, relax, and even to sleep, and their complex interactions rule your moods, whether up or down.

Neurotransmitters, or brain messengers, are made from proteins. Because of this, diet profoundly influences brain-messenger levels. Proteins that make up the brain messengers originate from a blend of different dietary amino acids. The gastrointestinal tract digests proteins into the smaller building blocks, the amino acids, that make up proteins. The amino acids are later reassembled into a number of proteins, including the brain messengers and proteins such as collagen, elastin, and chromosomes.

Tyrosine. Dopamine is one of the core brain messengers that maintain attention, motor coordination, sexual arousal, and a healthy immune system. The amino acid tyrosine is converted into dopa, the precursor of dopamine. Dopa is converted into dopamine only in the brain, since dopamine cannot cross the BrainGate. Dopamine can easily become depleted by stress, alcohol, caffeine, high-sugar diets, and lack of sleep. Oxidizing conditions inactivate dopamine, thus dietary antioxidants have a sparing effect on dopamine levels.

Norepinephrine is one of the main excitatory brain messengers used to stay alert or motivated, and it regulates the metabolic rate.

Healthy levels of norepinephrine are required to store new memories and fix them in the long-term memory banks. Norepinephrine and dopamine both use the amino acids tyrosine or phenylalanine as building materials. The generation of these brain messengers also requires vitamin C, B-family vitamins, and some copper and iron.

Good sources of tyrosine are avocados, almonds, bananas, lima beans, pumpkin seeds, and sesame seeds.

Tryptophan. Serotonin is a mood-enhancing brain messenger needed for proper sleep patterns. Serotonin plays other critical roles by influencing learning and memory. Low levels of serotonin can cause depression, insomnia, and obsessive-compulsive disorders. Serotonin is made from tryptophan but also needs B-family vitamins for the conversion.

Good sources of tryptophan are brown rice, peanuts, and sesame seeds.

Choline. Acetylcholine is an excitatory brain messenger needed for concentration, thinking, memory, and motor skills. Low levels of acetylcholine typically occur with advanced age and can lead directly to cognitive decline. Unlike the other primary brain messengers, acetylcholine is not manufactured from amino acids. Instead, this messenger is mostly made from the vitamin B-family choline. Once again, diet is critical here, since the more choline you eat the more acetylcholine your body will make. You can also obtain supplements of choline in the form of phosphatidylcholine. Vitamin C and vitamin B5 are needed for the acetylcholine conversion.

Good sources of choline are wheat germ, soybeans, and whole-wheat products.

Common Carbohydrates

Your car runs on gas; your brain runs on glucose. Many people know from personal experience that long periods of intense thought processes cause exhaustion. Mental exercise requires even more sleep to recover from than physical exercise. Because glucose provides one of the main sources of energy for the brain, mental tasks can quickly consume it. Research has demonstrated that prolonged, intensive mental activities can deplete glucose especially in the hippocampus, the region of the brain central to learning and memory function.

The research shows that a steady supply of glucose made available to the brain supports optimal cognitive functions. Rats subjected to maze tests showed plummeting glucose levels in the area of the hippocampus, resulting in declined thought processes, including memory formation and retrieval. The younger rats in the test supplied enough glucose to the brain until the mental task became very prolonged and difficult. The glucose depletion in the brain was more pronounced in older rats when they were subjected to identical mental tasks. Physiologists had previously believed that, except during starvation, the brain always found an adequate supply of glucose. The new experimental findings show that brain glucose supplies will fluctuate and that this fluctuation affects memory formation and learning tasks.

Steady supplies of glucose have the ability to enhance memory and learning in humans as well as rats. Optimal meals and proper meal timing, therefore, may bestow great benefits in terms of learning for people of all ages. When healthy older adults plagued with memory declines were given a memory test following a breakfast of barley and mashed potatoes, researchers discovered that the carbohydrates increased memory skills within one hour after the meal.

Other studies looked at healthy senior citizens who received a breakfast of cereal and grape juice, while another group received only water. When the groups were given a memory test twenty minutes later, the cereal-and-grape-juice group remembered test prompts about 25 percent better than those in the water-only group. A diet deficient in complex carbohydrates not only starves the brain of its main energy supply, it also impacts the levels of key brain messengers like acetylcholine.

The research found that complex carbohydrates provided superior long-term memory boosts when compared with both fats and proteins. The study stressed the importance of consuming complex carbohydrates in vegetables, fruits, and whole grains compared with the highly refined sugars found in processed foods.

Still other studies showed superior memory performance with complex carbohydrates compared with simple sugars. Those people who ate carbohydrate-laden breakfasts consisting of barley or potatoes displayed superior performance on both short-term and long-term memory tests compared with a group that drank lemon-flavored glucose drinks.

Low blood glucose levels can cause severe cognitive declines. The brain cells have very large energy demands—up to two times the energy requirements of other body cells. The brain uses electrical activity constantly, even during sleep. The most demanding energy task in the nervous system fuels the sodium and potassium membrane pumps that form the electrical potential (charge) used for the electric pulse that transmits brain signals. The membrane pump allows the electric signals to form and consumes about 50 percent of the total energy available to the brain.

We know glucose is used as the primary energy source by nerve cells. Since brain cells cannot store very much glucose, they depend on steady delivery from the BrainGate. Complex carbohydrates are digested slowly and supply a steady source of brain sugar.

High-simple-sugar foods (cookies, sodas) cause the blood sugar levels to spike, which, in turn, causes the pancreas to release insulin. Insulin facilitates sugar absorption in cells throughout the body. Often insulin will cause the blood sugar to plummet, making glucose available to the brain scarce and making you feel irritable, tired, weak, and unable to concentrate on mental activities.

To help alleviate dramatic swings in blood sugar, consume foods that have low glycemic indices. A glycemic index rates how quickly the carbohydrates enter the bloodstream. As you might guess, foods with the highest glycemic indices include the processed foods, such as instant rice, instant potatoes, and bleached white flour. Foods with low glycemic indices include whole fresh foods like barley; slow-cooked oatmeal; whole-grain products; fruits such as apples, grapes, and peaches; vegetables such as broccoli and cabbage. If you consume foods with high glycemic indices, make sure to combine them with low-glycemic-index foods, which will lower the glycemic index of the entire meal. For example, jelly has a high glycemic index and whole-grain bread has a lower glycemic index, yet, when eaten together, the combined foods have a lower glycemic index than expected.

People who consume large amounts of high-sugar soda drinks also tend to have low levels of a number of key vitamins and minerals. Diets high in soda deplete the body of magnesium, a mineral that participates in almost all of the key reactions required for nerve cells to generate energy for the brain. Magnesium assists in the conversion of fats into DHA, the brain's primary cell membrane fat. The brain also requires magnesium to make the myelin sheaths that cover and electrically insulate the nerves. Western diets consisting mainly of animal products provide poor sources of magnesium. In addition, processing or lengthy cooking of foods further strips them of magnesium.

Vitamins and Minerals

Researchers have found on a number of occasions that consuming whole fresh fruits and vegetables provides superior antioxidant protection versus taking vitamin pills. For example, researchers found that most of the antioxidant activity of apples results from the phytochemical content. Eating 100 grams of a fresh apple complete with the skin provides the same amount of antioxidant protection as 1,500 milligrams of vitamin C. These studies emphasize the often overlooked contribution of phytochemicals from fresh plant foods.

The use of vitamin supplements has spurred controversy. A number of researchers have gone on record to say that vitamin supplements merely waste money. Yet a large group of consumers fuel a multi-billion-dollar supplement market.

If you consume the ideal diet—fresh, organic, and plant-based—and live in a pollution-free environment, you likely won't need extra vitamins. But you don't live in your great-grandparents' world: today no one lives pollution-free! Further, with advancing age you just don't produce the amounts of brain-friendly fats, like DHA, as you did when you were younger. So selecting the appropriate nutritional supplements may help in lowering your risk of mental disorders.

How Do Vitamins Protect?

Specialized proteins called enzymes speed up chemical reactions. Human life would not exist without enzymes to accelerate life's chemical reactions. In order to work, many enzymes require other items called co-factors such as vitamins and minerals. Enzyme co-factors often act as growth-limiting factors and must be supplied in the diet. Even people who believe they eat a healthy diet usually show deficiencies in several vitamins and co-factors.

When enzymes have enough co-factors, further increasing vitamins or minerals will not further increase enzyme activity. Higher levels of vitamins reach a point at which they no longer produce further increases in enzyme activity. For this reason, many researchers have concluded that taking in more vitamins than you need is actually wasteful. But vitamins possess many other disease-preventing qualities. For example, vitamins such as C, E, folic acid, and beta-carotene halt the actions of some disease-causing chemicals, such as nitrosamines, and have powerful antioxidant activity.

When to Exceed the RDA for Vitamins

—If you are pregnant.

—If you eat an animal-based diet.

—If you consume mostly processed foods.

—If you take prescription drugs, painkillers, diuretics, laxatives, antibiotics, or birth control drugs.

—If you smoke cigarettes or use tobacco or alcohol.

—If you have diarrhea or other disorders of the digestive tract.

—If you drink caffeine or alcoholic beverages.

—If you are exposed to pollutants either at home or work.

Many vitamins reduce brain disease and cancer risks and have little toxicity, even when taken in quantities many times greater than the Recommended Daily Dietary Allowances (RDA). Most people have different lifestyles and various health ailments, or they reside in polluted environs and therefore require greater intakes of antioxidant vitamins.

Tobacco smoking increases risks of emotional disturbances, cancer, heart disease, and lung disease. Smokers have lower levels of many antioxidant vitamins—such as vitamin C, beta-carotene, and vitamin B6—than nonsmokers.

Teenagers have greater nutritional demands, but they also have poor eating habits that often don't meet vitamin requirements. Folic acid is deficient in about half of otherwise healthy teenage girls. Today the United States has record numbers of overweight teens, a problem caused by poor diets and widespread lack of exercise.

Weight-loss programs often limit entire food groups and can harm vitamin levels. People who remove all plant carbohydrates from their diet take in meager amounts of antioxidants, get less protection from fiber, and don't receive the sustained release of sugar for optimal brain activity. Supplements can take the place of diets that remove all animal foods that provide small amounts of vitamin B12. Without the use of supplements, however, it becomes very difficult to meet the vitamin requirements with most weight-loss diets.

Drug use blocks vitamin uptake and increases the requirement for more vitamins. Women taking birth control pills have lower levels of beta-carotene, vitamin B6, vitamin C, and folic acid. Many common antibiotics and antacids interfere with the uptake of vitamins. Aspirin and antiepilepsy drugs can interfere with the uptake of folic acid, and, if taken daily, will lead to vitamin deficiencies. Frequent use of alcohol also lowers the levels of vitamin D, beta-carotene, folic acid, thiamin, and vitamin B6.

Pregnancy places greater demands on the body's need for vitamins, especially during the critical first trimester of pregnancy. In many pregnancies, the mother has low levels of at least one vitamin at the time of birth. Older people also have vitamin deficiencies that can result from poor diets, dental conditions, and other illnesses. Older people may also have reduced capacity for digesting and absorbing some vitamins.

Vitamin A

Studies reveal that vitamin A plays a vital role in the brain, visual processes, and growth of skin. The liver stores most of the vitamin A in the body. People with proper diets can store enough vitamin A to last for months. Symptoms of vitamin A deficiency include night blindness, increased lung infections, and dry, rough skin.

Vitamin A may prevent brain disease in several ways. Vitamin A encourages the growth and maintenance of surface cells, or epithelial tissues, where many brain disorders can arise. Vitamin A also plays a critical role in the immune system by blocking tumor cell growth.

Dietary sources of vitamin A include asparagus, broccoli, carrots, peas, and pumpkins. Beta-carotene, found in deep-yellow and dark-green vegetables, is converted to vitamin A. The RDA for vitamin A for adults is 5,000 IU. Vitamin A is toxic if consumed at high doses. Do not increase the intake beyond the RDA for vitamin A. Pregnant women need to use special caution with vitamin A, since in very large doses it causes birth defects.

Health Benefits of Vitamin A

—Supports brain health and nervous tissues

—Reduces strokes and cancer risks

—Increases the immune response

—Helps maintain healthy skin

Beta-Carotene

Beta-carotene belongs to a family of over six hundred yellow, orange, and red plant pigments. Beta-carotene is critical for brain health and cancer prevention. The body converts beta-carotene into vitamin A, and some believe vitamin A actually provides the protection rather than beta-carotene. Current research shows beta-carotene can provide protection independently from vitamin A.

Vision-impairing cataracts can result from clouding in the lens of the eye during periods of low antioxidant levels. People with poor beta-carotene levels exhibit about a six times greater chance of developing cataracts. The lens of the eye contains very small amounts of beta-carotene; therefore, beta-carotene may prevent cataracts by sparing other antioxidant vitamins that serve to protect the lens.

Beta-carotene is basically nontoxic. The body converts only the required amounts of vitamin A from beta-carotene, and large intakes of beta-carotene do not result in high levels of vitamin A. Very high intakes of beta-carotene can result in a reversible yellow coloring of the skin.

Health Benefits of Beta-Carotene

—Protects against development of cataracts
—Protects the brain through antioxidant properties
—Improves the immune system
—Protects in light-sensitive skin disorders
—Protects from cancers
—Protects tobacco users

The B vitamins act as co-factors used to produce energy in the brain. Studies show that elderly people deficient in either vitamin B12 or folic acid were two times more likely to come down with Alzheimer's when compared with a group who had normal B vitamin levels. Both B12 and folic acid are vital to healthy mental function. People of advanced age have a greater risk of malnutrition. The researchers stressed that no evidence exists that the vitamin deficiencies caused Alzheimer's disease.

Many people have B12 deficiencies. Nearly two out of five people tested have vitamin B12 levels low enough to display the typical deficiency symptoms such as less sensation in their limbs, and memory and balance problems. Serious B12 depletion can lead to nerve cell damage and dementia. Most B-family vitamins are soluble in water and don't stay in the body long; therefore, we need constant supplies from the diet.

Good sources for B-vitamins include whole grains, beans, fresh leafy green vegetables, wheat germ, and brewer's yeast. High-temperature cooking or commercial food-processing destroys many of the B-family vitamins.

Vitamin B1 (Thiamin)

Vitamin B1 (or thiamin) helps produce the myelin sheath that covers nerves like insulation on a wire and allows nerve signals to pass. Thiamin also encourages the general health and functioning of the nervous system and helps maintain proper mental health. Thiamin supports the conversion of glucose into useable energy. If a marginal thiamin deficiency exists, nerves degenerate and overreact to stimuli, making a person easily irritated and forgetful.

Vitamin B2 (Riboflavin)

Vitamin B2 (or riboflavin) also assists in the production of energy. Riboflavin has been shown to decrease the frequency and duration of migraine headaches. Researchers concluded that riboflavin recipients boosted specific energy-producing areas of the brain involved in triggering a migraine. The riboflavin prevented a low-energy state, which may explain how it prevents migraines.

Vitamin B3 (Niacin)

Vitamin B3 (niacin or nicotinic acid) is also a required co-factor in many processes, including energy production. Niacin assists the power generator (mitochondria) to make energy. Good sources of niacin include whole grains and peanuts. The RDA for niacin is 20 milligrams per day for adults.

Vitamin B12

Vitamin B12 is needed to make amino acids, fats, and DNA. Poor levels of vitamin B12 can cause irreversible nervous system damage.

Vitamin B12 sources include foods of animal origin. A variety of B-family supplements also include B12. Vitamin B12 has few side effects, even in doses higher than the RDA. The RDA for vitamin B12 is 6 micrograms per day.

Folic Acid

Folic acid is a required co-factor for a number of enzymes that make DNA. For proper infant brain growth during pregnancy, mothers need folic acid. Failed closings of the neural tube that later becomes the spinal cord, a condition known as spina bifida, can result from folic acid deficiency during pregnancy. Folic acid also converts the toxic amino acid homocysteine to methionine. Folic acid will lower the homocysteine levels, particularly in people with very high homocysteine. The conversion is vital to keeping a healthy brain and heart, and buildup of homocysteine is toxic. Folic acid is relatively nontoxic and safe even when intake is very high. Alcohol, birth control pills, and drugs used to treat convulsions all lower folic acid levels. Folic acid also needs B6, B12, magnesium, and biotin for converting homocysteine into methionine. A poor intake of either vitamin B6 or B12 will also result in elevated homocysteine levels.

Vegetables, especially dark-green leafy vegetables, fresh fruits, lentils,

Health Benefits of Folic Acid

—Increases memory in older individuals
—Helps to decrease homocysteine, which causes aggression and heart disease risk
—Prevents neural tube and cleft palate defects
—Is required for DNA manufacture and repair
—Is critical for a healthy heart and blood vessels
—Prevents chromosome defects
—Reduces risk of uterine, cervix, intestine, colon, and lung cancers

Food Sources for Folic Acid

—Dark-green leafy vegetables, especially collard greens, spinach, romaine lettuce, Brussels sprouts, beets
—Lentils and soybeans
—Fresh fruits and vegetables, especially oranges and grapefruit, asparagus, peas, avocados, broccoli, and okra
—Navy beans
—Nuts
—Whole-wheat products; wheat germ; bulgur

soybeans, nuts, beans, and yeast are good sources of folic acid. High-temperature cooking or commercial food-processing (canning) will destroy folic acid. The RDA of folic acid for adults is 400 micrograms per day, and for pregnant women, 800 micrograms per day.

Vitamin C

Vitamin C is very important to the brain, since the brain concentrates vitamin C up to 100 times higher than other tissues. When vitamin C levels drop in the brain, it gets shuttled into the brain from other parts of the body. Vitamin C participates in making the brain messengers dopamine and norepinephrine. Researchers generally place vitamin C at the center of the antioxidant defense hub.

In Finland, a study that investigated smokers tested the efficacy of beta-carotene in preventing lung cancer. Surprisingly, the smokers given beta-carotene actually displayed a higher level of lung cancer. This result isn't that unusual when you consider that vitamin C reduces oxidized and inactive vitamin E and beta-carotene back to their active, reduced forms. If you give extra beta-carotene, you also need extra vitamin C. Therefore, the strength of beta-carotene's antioxidant power depends on the simultaneous presence of vitamin C. Antioxidant vitamins act in concert or synergy with one another providing even greater protection.

The Finnish study also demonstrates the complexity of nutritional studies that go against the scientific methods that change as few variables as possible. Scientists prefer to study only one to three variables in a study. But you cannot examine only one antioxidant in isolation from the others when they work in interconnected manners. Therefore, the scientific dogma of investigating small numbers of variables can fail us when the elements of nutrition depend entirely on one another.

Vitamin C is an antioxidant that keeps free radicals in check and limits the damage to cell components. Vitamin C assists in making collagen, the most common protein in the body. Collagen is also a critical part of skin, cartilage, tendons, ligaments, bones, teeth, and

Health Benefits of Vitamin C

- —Promotes mental acuity (mild vitamin C deficiency can lead to mental confusion and depression)
- —Promotes wound healing (people with poor vitamin C intake bruise easily, and have slow wound healing)
- —Promotes the integrity of the BrainGate by encouraging collagen and elastin growth
- —Decreases genetic damage in people exposed to DNA-harming chemicals
- —Reduces risk of oral, throat, stomach, colon, rectal, cervical, and pancreatic cancers
- —Promotes resistance to infection by forming stronger collagen, providing a better physical barrier from bacteria, viruses, and tumor cells
- —Reduces stroke risk
- —Acts as an antioxidant, protecting the brain
- —Blocks formation of cancer-causing chemicals like nitrosamines
- —Improves cardiovascular health (may lower blood pressure)
- —Prevents cataract formation
- —Enhances liver clearance of toxic chemicals
- —Reduces the toxicity of some pollutants like pesticides, heavy metals, hydrocarbons, ozone, and carbon monoxide
- —Enhances the immune system

blood vessels. Collagen forms the underlying structural framework for connective tissue in the BrainGate. Without sufficient vitamin C, the collagen produced is weak and easily broken down. If this weakened collagen is taken up into the brain, the integrity of the BrainGate could be compromised and may leak more than normal. Vitamin C is also required to produce elastin, a connective tissue that gives skin and blood vessels their elastic nature to help keep pulse pressure low.

Vitamin C may prevent brain disease and cancers through its antioxidant properties, by decreasing the formation of toxic nitrosamines, by enhancing the immune system, and by detoxifying certain toxic chemicals. In human studies, vitamin C dramatically decreased levels of nitrosamines that may cause brain cancer. High levels of vitamin C may also reduce the risk of digestive tract (oral, throat, stomach, colon, and rectal) cancers. Vitamin C may also protect from lung and cervix cancers and cancer of the pancreas.

Vitamin C supports the immune system by enhancing the function of white blood cells. Like vitamin E, vitamin C helps to prevent strokes that cause declines in brain function. Vitamin C also reduces the risk of cataracts. In one study, those who did not receive vitamin C (300 to 600 mg/day) had a fourfold greater chance of forming cataracts.

Strawberries, Brussels sprouts, tomatoes, artichokes, citrus fruits, rose hips, black currants, guava, cranberries, kale, parsley, peppers, broccoli, collards, and cabbage all contain vitamin C. High-temperature cooking and the processing of food depletes vitamin C, and dried fruits have lost most of their vitamin C content. People exposed to smog, environmental chemicals, or cigarette smoke require more vitamin C. Stress depletes vitamin C, since stress hormones use vitamin C as a raw product in the manufacture of stress hormones. Vitamin C has few toxic side effects except diarrhea, which occurs if the vitamin is taken in extreme doses. The RDA for vitamin C is 60 mg/day.

Vitamin E

Vitamin E is fat-soluble and helps to protect brain cell membranes. Since cell membranes contain polyunsaturated fats, they easily oxidize in a way similar to butter turning rancid. Vitamin E protects membranes from this rancidity. Fat tissue, liver, and muscle primarily store vitamin E, but with high intakes all tissues will store vitamin E. The RDA for vitamin E is 30 IU. Wheat germ oil, wheat bran, legumes, vegetable oils, nuts, seeds, and green plants provide rich sources of vitamin E.

Vitamin E and C act together to block the conversion of the nitrates (from fertilizer) into nitrosamines that damage DNA and may cause brain and other cancers.

When injured, blood vessels spill blood. Small rod-like cells, called platelets, stick to the damaged site and eventually block further blood loss. An exaggerated platelet response, however, will increase the chance of a heart attack or brain stroke. Diets high in the pro-inflammatory omega-6 fats also increase the risk of forming blood clots. Vitamin E encourages the platelets not to respond too eagerly and decreases the risk of strokes. Vitamin E content in platelets declines with advancing age, and platelets with less vitamin E clump together more easily. Vitamin E lowers the risk of brain strokes in individuals who have rich diets of vitamin E. Less risk from heart disease has also been shown with intakes of at least 300 mg of vitamin E per day.

People with brain disorders like Alzheimer's and Parkinson's disease exhibit more deficiencies in vitamin E. Vitamin E stabilizes and protects membranes by providing antioxidant protection. Nervous tissue such as the brain is particularly susceptible to oxidative damage. Environmental pollutants can play a role in brain diseases and vitamin E helps in their prevention. Vitamin E works together with selenium and increases the antioxidant potential. Selenium, a trace mineral, also acts as a co-factor in antioxidant enzymes that detoxify free radicals.

Walnuts, almonds, soybeans, and unrefined expeller(cold)-pressed oils contain high levels of vitamin E. Wheat germ, brown rice, and oats provide good levels of vitamin E, and dark-green leafy vegetables, Brussels sprouts, and broccoli contain fair amounts.

Even at very high doses, vitamin E has few toxic side effects. Vitamin E can increase the blood-clotting times in people with certain diseases or with vitamin K deficiencies. However, people taking blood-thinning drugs (anticoagulants) should avoid high vitamin E intakes.

Health Benefits of Vitamin E

—Improves brain disorders such as Alzheimer's and Parkinson's
—Antioxidant properties help to repair and protect the brain cells and cell membranes
—Helps prevent heart disease, which in turn affects brain function
—Helps to keep blood-clotting activities in check and may help prevent brain strokes
—Protects from exposures to alcohol, smog, and tobacco
—Enhances the immune system
—Helps lower risk for gut, lung, breast, prostate, and throat cancers
—Helps with DNA repair
—Blocks nitrosamine formation, which is linked to brain cancer

Essential Minerals

Essential minerals play vital roles in brain health and, like vitamins, function as co-factors in the reactions necessary for life. Studies show that organically grown produce contains more minerals and trace elements than commercially grown produce.

If you think you have a deficiency in essential or trace metals or have been exposed to heavy metals, a metal analysis of your hair may provide a starting point to semiquantify your exposure levels. (A company that specializes in trace metal analysis of hair samples is listed in the Appendix.)

Exciting information reveals how olive oil diets make people less vulnerable to developing Alzheimer's and other age-related memory problems. Foods like mashed potatoes and barley have the power to improve memory minutes after consumption. These common carbohydrates particularly help the elderly and people with poor memories. By consuming the proper vitamins, fats, and foods that keep minerals in balance, you can enjoy optimal brain functions and even avoid the uptake of select toxic agents.

o

Food Sources of Essential Minerals

Boron	Garlic and onions
Calcium	Dark-green leafy vegetables; also widely distributed in dairy products, but not a recommended source
Chromium	Black pepper, broccoli, prunes, raisins, nuts, asparagus, brewer's yeast, beer, wine, wheat, wheat germ
Copper	Asparagus, nuts, whole-grain cereal, raisins, apples, broccoli
Fluorine	Spinach, peas, beets, whole-wheat bread, sweet potatoes
Germanium	Garlic and onions
Iodine	Seaweed, iodized salt
Iron	Blackstrap molasses, potatoes, kidney beans, tofu, dark-green vegetables, fruits, cereals; also widely distributed in red meat, but not a recommended source
Lithium	Tomatoes, mushrooms, cucumbers, red cabbage, black tea, paprika, marjoram
Magnesium	Nuts, legumes, cereal grains, chocolate, green vegetables, potatoes
Manganese	Avocados, unrefined cereals, dark bread, tea, ginger, nuts, seeds, beets, turnip greens, green leafy vegetables

(continued on next page)

Food Sources of Essential Minerals

(continued from previous page)

Molybdenum	Legumes, cereal, yeast
Nickel	Oats, cabbage
Phosphorus	Seeds, nuts, legumes, grains
Potassium	Vegetables, cabbage, spinach, molasses, peas, bananas, fruit, bran flakes, cocoa
Selenium	Cereals, garlic, Brazil nuts, seafood, wheat bran, soybeans, yeast
Silicon	Unrefined grains, oats, wheat bran, soybeans, beets, leafy vegetables, brown rice
Tin	Fruits, vegetables, juices
Vanadium	Green beans, whole grains, radishes
Zinc	Whole-grain products, nuts, seeds, green leafy vegetables

6

Eat to Beat the Blues

DEPRESSION, AMERICA'S MOST COMMON mental health problem, affects over 17 million people at some period in their lives. Consumers spend over $3 billion a year on depression-fighting drugs that target either serotonin or norepinephrine. Serotonin and norepinephrine are called neurotransmitters, since they transmit messages into brain cells. But for our purposes, we will call them brain messengers.

The number of people developing depression seems to have escalated in recent decades. And it is not surprising that more people are being prescribed antidepressant drugs. According to a new study, more people are relying on antidepressant drugs than psychotherapy to combat depression and anxiety. From 1987 to 1997, the number of depressed individuals using antidepressant drugs increased from about 37 percent to 75 percent, while those seeking psychotherapy decreased about 10 percent during the same period. Sexual dysfunction, a troublesome side effect of antidepressant drugs, is reported by 40 percent of people who use them. Although the drugs assist many depressed people, in about 20 percent of the cases they don't work.

Yet despite this increase in antidepressant prescriptions, many suffering from depression search for methods other than drugs to treat their condition. One strategy gaining popularity is the use of food choices and nutrition to lift mood. A large amount of evidence shows that food choices can profoundly influence moods.

For hundreds of thousands of years humans gathered and cultivated nuts, grains, fruits, and vegetables. Whole foods were a dietary staple, since food processing did not blossom until about the beginning of the twentieth century. Whole-food diets present a steady supply of various amino acids to the BrainGate. Once in the brain, these assorted amino acids are converted into brain messengers. Grains were likely the first foods to be processed by roller milling. Commercial processing of foods has exploded in the last half-century. We will discover how the BrainGate and processed foods play central roles in mental health and depression.

Unlocking the BrainGate

Understanding the complex roles of brain messengers helps us fight depression by guiding our food choices. Some foods truly are "food for thought."

Here's how it works. Brain messengers find receptors formed from protein complexes embedded into the surfaces of nerve cells. These receptors act like padlocks, since they only accept the correct key carried by particular brain messengers. The keys have the right shape and electrical properties that allow them entry into the padlock to open it.

Padlock (Receptor) and Brain Messenger

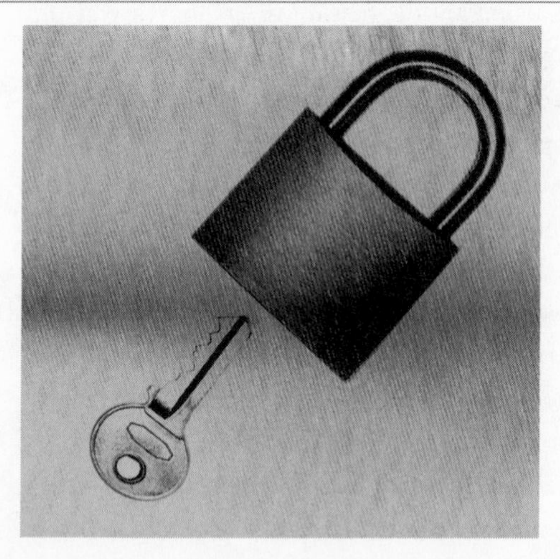

This interaction of the brain messengers and padlocks forms the basic core of information exchange through the entire nervous system. It allows for the efficient flow of data between individual brain cells, and it directs every thought and behavior. When a brain messenger attaches and unlocks a receptor padlock, it sends a signal into that brain cell. Imagine a key that occupies the keyhole of the padlock. When the key turns it also turns the padlocks tumblers, transferring a signal to the brain cell via the padlock, which in turn directs the cell to respond.

There are as many varieties of padlocks as there are brain messengers, and there are hundreds of padlock types for a specific brain messenger.

Even though each padlock is designed to be unlocked by a specific brain messenger, some drugs and plant chemicals can also unlock certain padlocks. So it's clear that many ingested substances can profoundly affect the nervous system.

These plant chemicals and drugs can act just like brain messengers and generate identical responses, or they might just occupy the padlock site and not allow the real brain messengers access, thereby blocking the normal response. Some toxic and addictive agents such as cocaine behave in this fashion.

The real problems have developed in the last half-century, as food processing has taken our food apart piece by piece. Food purveyors have transformed our diet into something that does not resemble whole food any more than bleached white flour bears a likeness to amber waves of grain.

A Body Out of Balance

When you consume whole foods, your digestive system slowly releases nutrients and makes them available to the blood and, hence, to the brain. Whole plant foods are assembled with complex carbohydrates, the long chains of sugar molecules that your liver slowly digests into simple glucose molecules to fuel the brain. Plant foods also contain fiber (cellulose), which resists digestion and further slows sugar uptake into the blood. Glucose is gradually released by the gut lining to the liver, which stores and releases it as needed to keep a steady supply for the brain. The natural plant foods work like time-release vitamins, slowly releasing glucose over long periods of time.

When you eat highly processed foods, however, specific amino acids and simple sugars, added only to enhance taste, rush into the blood. The BrainGate is flooded with these added flavor-enhancing amino acids. At first blush, this condition might not seem so bad, except that it prevents the transport of many other amino acids necessary for optimal brain health. (Imagine people swarming the turnstile gates while entering a baseball park when an emergency crew needs to enter.)

In addition, if you consume animal protein, the large neutral amino acids will clog the turnstile that tryptophan uses to cross into the brain. When the brain is deprived of tryptophan, it can't produce enough serotonin to have a calming influence. In fact, the major class of antidepressant drugs acts by slowing the removal of serotonin and effectively increasing its levels in the brain.

Furthermore, when you eat processed foods, excess sugar absorbed into the blood triggers a massive release of insulin. Insulin encourages the cells to absorb glucose (except brain cells), so glucose levels can plummet to the point where low blood sugar or hypoglycemia results. Researchers have discovered a trend in people with low blood sugar: they tend to be more irritated, showing aggression and depression. Therefore, two simple components of food, sugars and amino acids, can act alone or together to dramatically influence your moods.

Foods to Rev You Up or Calm You Down

Since the assorted brain messengers are made in brain cells, their manufacture is completely dependent upon what types of amino acids actually cross into the brain. Because of the brain's protective BrainGate, the uptake of amino acids is a bit complex (see Chapter 1). Recall that the BrainGate prevents many things you eat from gaining access to your brain cells.

To arrive at brain cells, amino acids must first cross the BrainGate. The amino acids have to be escorted across the BrainGate by a shuttle that requires fuel. Amino acids in the same family have to use a limited number of specific shuttle vehicles. Since they have to compete for shuttle space to cross the BrainGate into the brain, diet directly affects the specific types of amino acids that are shuttled into the brain.

For example, the amino acids tryptophan and tyrosine both pass the BrainGate in the same shuttle vehicle. If your diet is rich in tryptophan, your blood levels will be high and your brain cells will get more tryptophan to convert into the calming serotonin. On the other hand, if your diet is rich in tyrosine, your brain will produce more norepinephrine and dopamine, two brain messengers that excite and contribute to increased physical activity and mental alertness.

Milk contains tryptophan, but drinking milk actually decreases the brain's uptake of tryptophan because of the presence of other amino acids such as tyrosine, valine, and leucine, which crowd the transport shuttle, much like what happens at that ballpark turnstile before a game.

High-carbohydrate diets can elevate the brain's tryptophan levels, and increase the levels of serotonin. It makes sense, then, that a carbohydrate-rich meal might be more appealing for the late evening snack and dinner.

In contrast, proteins might make more sense in the morning, since they elevate tyrosine levels in the blood, so the brain produces more norepinephrine and dopamine. Tyrosine is critical to brain activity and mental alertness in other ways. The thyroid uses tyrosine to produce active hormones to regulate metabolism for optimal brain health. Hence low dietary intake and low blood levels of tyrosine relate to underactive thyroid glands and sluggish physical activity.

The Brain in Balance

As with many things in life, it's best to have balance, and this is especially true with nutrition. When you consume a range of whole foods that contain a mixture of amino acids, your brain will use these to produce a balance of energizing and calming brain messengers. In contrast, if your diet is heavy in animal products and processed foods, you could very well skew the mixture of amino acids in a depressing direction.

Many processed foods contain additives like MSG or large amounts of one particular amino acid that will send your amino acids out of balance. You might also think twice about consuming foods that contain the artificial sweetener aspartame. Aspartame has been found to disrupt the uptake and balance of amino acids in the brain. One amino acid in particular, phenylalanine, becomes elevated in blood, which parallels a rise in the brain. This can be damaging because phenylalanine can compete with tryptophan for shuttle transport through the BrainGate and disrupt the production of brain messengers.

Whole fresh foods provide the most suitable source for dietary amino acids. Think carefully before eating amino acids in tablet or liquid forms, however, since these can have potent effects on the type of amino acids crossing the BrainGate. Optimal brain nutrition will assist in maintaining the balance of brain messenger levels. Other factors can also affect brain messenger levels, such as infections, stress hormones, poor circulation (heart and vascular disease), and gut ailments.

Note: It's important to obtain your tryptophan from whole foods and not from supplements. In 1989 about five thousand people suffered from a disease called eosinophilic myalgia syndrome. The disease caused permanent nervous system damage and was eventually traced to a toxic contaminant found in tryptophan supplements. As a result, the FDA has banned the sale of tryptophan supplements.

Food Sources of Important Amino Acids

Tyrosine	Tryptophan	Serotonin
Almonds, avocados, bananas, lima beans, pumpkin seeds, sesame seeds, soybeans, sunflower seeds, peanuts	Barley, brown rice, fish, soybeans, peanuts, sesame seeds, sunflower seeds, lentils, peas, pumpkins, kelp, algae	Bananas, plantains, tomatoes, red plums, purple plums, avocados, pineapples, passion fruit

You can obtain the metabolite of tryptophan (5-HTP) as a supplement, yet it is unclear whether 5-HTP is safe or effective.

Natural Highs

A number of other foods and nutrients have also been shown to alter moods. These include essential fatty acids like DHA, carbohydrates, spicy foods, garlic, caffeine, and foods rich in tryptophan, selenium, and folic acid.

Bleak moods may result from a simple nutritional deficiency. If you suffer from depression, the first course of action is to investigate the nutritional balance of your diet. Changing your diet has far fewer side effects than taking antidepressant drugs. A number of studies show that a diet poor in folic acid can lead not only to depression, but—if the deficiency is severe—also to dementia and schizophrenia. When folic acid levels were corrected in the studies, so was most of the depression. Good whole-food sources of folic acid include dark-green leafy vegetables like spinach; lentils; soybeans; nuts; beans; fresh fruits and vegetables; and yeast.

Selenium is another micronutrient associated with positive moods. Studies have shown that people consuming low amounts of selenium in their diet are more apt to suffer from gloomy moods. Good food sources of selenium are whole grains such as oats and wheat, and Brazil nuts and sunflower seeds.

Spicy foods—especially those high in chili peppers—can cause a release of endorphins (the brain compounds that cause "runners' high"). Endorphins can give you a temporary sense of wellness and a great mental boost.

Investigators who looked at garlic's effects on lowering cholesterol discovered, to their surprise, that garlic also increased the mood of the study participants. The garlic-receiving group reported much higher levels of energy and less anxiety and irritability.

Another natural treatment for depression is S-adenosylmethionine (SAM). The theory is that SAM increases the production of brain messengers such as serotonin and perhaps norepinephrine. However, there is some evidence to suggest that SAM is poorly absorbed from oral routes and therefore may not be effective to treat depression.

Fats to Fight Depression and Improve Cognition

Essential brain fat levels are also linked to healthy cognition. Processed foods are poor sources of essential fats and may even contain toxic and chemically altered fats.

Scientists have related the rising rates of depression in North America during the last century to the declining levels of essential fats such as DHA in our diets. In addition to the high stresses modern life contributes to increased depression, researchers stated that the "relative deficiencies in essential fatty acids may also intensify vulnerability to depression."

Researchers noted that fewer cases of major depression were found in areas of the world where the diet is rich in DHA. Furthermore, North American and European populations showed combined rates of depression that were 10 times greater than a Taiwanese group that ate a diet rich in fish. The Japanese, whose traditional diet includes fish, have dramatically lower rates of depression compared with North Americans and Europeans. However, fish is not a recommended source of DHA; Neuromins is preferred (see Appendix). Finally, researchers have discovered that seriously depressed patients had lower DHA levels than mildly depressed patients.

Protein

How Protein Consumption Affects Your Mood

For many generations now, Americans have been constantly reminded about getting enough protein. Consuming "enough protein" is so ingrained in our American way of thinking that most of us routinely consume animal proteins—some form of meat, dairy, or poultry—at every meal.

The notion that animal protein is superior to plant protein appears to originate from a study conducted in 1914, when researchers investigated the protein requirements of rats. The study demonstrated that rats grew quicker when fed animal proteins than when they consumed plant proteins. Now, certainly, a rat is very different from a human, and it is reasonable to have some skepticism whenever you relate data from one species to another. Regardless, the researchers used the study results and classified animal protein, consisting of eggs, meat, and dairy products, as "Class A" proteins. Plant proteins were relegated to "Class B" proteins. The concept of proteins being classified differently if they originated from plants or animals was eliminated from use in England in 1959, but not in the United States, where powerful marketing forces still perpetuate the animal protein myth.

It's not surprising that not all scientists agree on an exact amount of daily protein requirements for human needs. Scientific literature places the number somewhere between 2 percent and 8 percent of the total diet. These protein percentages have an added safety margin, so the recommended dietary allowances are more than sufficient for 98 percent of the population.

So How Much Protein Do We Need?

What are human dietary protein requirements? Probably a lot less than most people believe. The protein content of mothers' milk provides an estimate of the upper level of protein needs, since newborn children grow more rapidly than at any other period in their life. Rat milk contains about 49 percent protein and cow's milk is 15 percent protein. It is very interesting that human breast milk only contains about 5 percent protein. This reduced level shows that humans have much lower protein needs than many other animals.

To this day, the dairy industry presses consumers with false claims about the benefits of consuming three glasses of milk per day, and meat producers market the "exclusive" protein benefits of a meat-based diet. Ironically, if we dined on potatoes alone, which contain about 11 percent protein, we would obtain enough protein for our body's needs.

No one suggests that you eat only potatoes, but nutritionists agree that plant protein is a very appropriate source of protein and that it's hard *not* to receive an adequate amount of calories and proteins while consuming a plant-based diet.

Excess Protein in the Human Diet

Contrary to general belief, little or no clear evidence shows that even intense physical exercise elevates your dietary protein requirements. The truth is, there are no health advantages to eating more protein than is required. In fact, consuming more protein than necessary can actually harm your health.

Take the kidneys, the organs responsible for processing excess protein, for example. High protein intake puts you at greater risk for developing kidney stones, kidney degeneration, and inflammation compared with proper levels of dietary protein. Researchers generally agree on the association between excess animal protein and an increased risk for osteoporosis. In fact, the most important risk factor for osteoporosis is the excess intake of protein.

Excess animal protein consumption is associated with osteoporosis, kidney disease, cancer, decreased serotonin production, and heightened levels of aggression and violence.

High Dietary Protein Lowers Serotonin and Causes Aggression and Obsessive-Compulsive Disorder

Excess dietary protein not only weakens your bones, it may also increase aggression. Proteins are made from amino acids, and since they are digested into amino acids they also influence moods.

The brain messenger serotonin creates a sense of wellness and is also needed for proper sleep. When serotonin levels are low, depression is more likely to occur.

Serotonin keys fit about fifteen padlocks in the body. When a person reaches the age of about twenty, one of the most common serotonin padlocks begins to disappear from the brain. This padlock (identified by scientists as 5-HT2A) was shown to decline about 15 percent per decade, and may explain why depression more commonly surfaces in middle age. Depression also seems more likely to occur in middle-aged people with animal-protein–based diets.

When researchers examined the brains of healthy men and women twenty to seventy years old, they discovered significant age-related declines in the number of these serotonin padlocks (5-HT2A) in the brain. The losses were more severe in the prefrontal cortex and hippocampus of the brain. Surprisingly, at the time, none of the study subjects suffered from depression. Researchers have also observed that padlocks for the brain messenger dopamine also diminish with advancing age.

We know that the human body converts certain dietary components into specific brain messengers. We know that tryptophan in particular converts into the brain messenger serotonin. We also know that serotonin is a critical brain messenger that imparts a calming influence and decreases the impulses toward violence and aggression. Most animal proteins consumed in the American diet are composed of many amino acids other than tryptophan. Thus, a high-animal-protein meal floods the BrainGate with large (neutral) amino acids that compete for transport into the brain, edging out tryptophan and reducing the amount of it that gets into the brain. The less dietary tryptophan, the less serotonin will be made. The less serotonin, the greater the impulses toward aggressive action, anger, and violence.

Since serotonin also functions to regulate mood, appetite, and impulse control, its levels are also linked with eating disorders associated with obsessive-compulsive disorders (OCDs). Some OCD-related eating disorders may be related to abnormally low levels of serotonin. To help the brain increase serotonin levels, drugs known to raise serotonin were administered to a group of people suffering from OCD. The treated subjects significantly reduced their OCD-related repetitive movements, experienced a dramatic drop in thoughts of suicide, and functioned better at school and work.

Carbohydrates

Can You Control Your Mood with Carbohydrates?

Many people who feel tired or perhaps a bit down in the late afternoon often reach for a starchy carbohydrate or some other source of sugar for quick energy. Most believe that an increase in blood glucose will make them more alert and provide a mental boost. It is true that glucose will increase your alertness—but only up to a point. Complex carbohydrates—those found in plants—are slowly digested and converted by the liver into glucose. On the other hand, high-sugar snack foods cause a rapid rise and fall of the blood sugar.

A number of studies have looked at the effects of carbohydrate on moods. It seems a small burst in energy follows a sugary snack, but that burst is followed by a feeling of sleepiness about two hours later. The studies also found that carbohydrates seem to have a greater relaxing and sedative effect and directly alter moods more than protein-rich meals. Blood glucose levels can also affect someone's mood much more critically when the person is under stress.

Glucose Levels and Mood Under Stress

Most studies have looked at blood glucose levels and the moods of unstressed subjects. Far fewer studies have explored how proper blood glucose levels maintain positive moods during mental challenges. Because the brain hungers for glucose, it makes sense that rising and falling supplies of glucose will alter moods, especially while one is performing demanding mental activities.

In one such study, researchers in the United Kingdom measured subjects' moods before and after undergoing three mentally challenging tests. In all three mental tasks, the subjects with persistently low blood glucose reported less energy and more tension or anxiety than those whose blood glucose was higher.

Gloomy states of mind or moods also occur with the low blood glucose typical of diabetics, whereas positive moods tend to be related to high blood glucose.

Sugar and Depression

A fair amount of evidence shows that picking the right carbohydrates can relieve depression. We know that low brain levels of serotonin are linked with depression and anxiety. And complex carbohydrate intake coupled with low protein intake has been shown to enhance serotonin production. A study showed that those who ate high-carbohydrate meals felt less depressed and more alert. The subjects who did not eat carbohydrates felt more sleepy and fatigued.

People afflicted with seasonal affective disorder (SAD) tend to eat more and gain weight in the winter seasons. Researchers have also found that eating high-carbohydrate, low-protein meals was associated with improved moods in people suffering from seasonal affective disorder. Many women experience premenstrual syndrome as they cycle through their menstrual periods. Researchers discovered that a high-carbohydrate meal improved the mood of women with premenstrual syndrome; anger, confusion, depression, and tension lessened or resolved after high carbohydrate intake.

Plant Carbohydrates As Part of the Daily Diet

When female cyclists were given diets consisting of either low, medium, or high levels of carbohydrate for one week, the cyclists who consumed the low-carbohydrate diet experienced increased anger, depression, and tension . Other studies have supported this trend. One group of subjects who were fed a low-carbohydrate and high-protein breakfast for three consecutive weeks showed increased levels of anger. A consistent trend shows that consuming a diet high in carbohydrates and low in protein is linked with better moods.

Researchers have also shown that a high-carbohydrate meal elevates the level of tryptophan compared with other large neutral amino acids such as leucine, isoleucine, tyrosine, phenylalanine, and valine.

Glucose and Aggression

It is also commonly accepted that low blood sugar will make you more aggressive and irritable. We know that someone who ingests a high amount of refined sugar will have a rapid increase in blood glucose that triggers an exaggerated release of insulin, which causes blood glucose to fall to an even lower level, thus depriving the brain of its steady supply of glucose.

Research in Finland shows that violent criminals have a unique pattern of rising and falling blood glucose. Prisoners who had committed violent crimes were given a glucose tolerance test, which determines how blood glucose levels react to an additional dose of glucose. After the glucose dose, the prisoners' glucose levels increased to abnormally high levels and shortly plummeted to a particularly low blood level. Hours later, the blood glucose very slowly returned to the pre–glucose-challenge levels. Another violent population is the Quolla Indians, who inhabit the high altitudes in Peru and are infamous for their high murder rate and family conflicts. Not surprisingly, most researchers have examined the Quolla's violent culture purely from their sociological roots. Yet research that measured glucose levels in the Quolla discovered that the most aggressive individuals tended to have blood glucose levels that plummeted to very low levels after they were given a glucose challenge.

Researchers have also monitored insulin secretion. They found that many violent criminals have an exaggerated insulin release in response to high blood glucose. Higher-than-normal amounts of insulin are released, which results in rapidly falling blood glucose levels. It is interesting that the tendency to develop low blood sugar is also a trait of people with antisocial personalities.

In another study, healthy six- or seven-year-old children were studied to find out how they would respond to failure while playing a computer game. The children who received a glucose drink were much less likely to respond with signs of frustration when compared with children who received the placebo.

Therefore, it seems that individuals whose blood glucose falls quicker in response to high sugar intake may be prone to irritability and may even display more aggression. A distinct possibility also exists that other factors such as a hormone may trigger aggression during times of low blood glucose.

Typical sodas and other soft drinks have hyperconcentrated sugar loads—so high that the sugar would convert from liquid to crystallized sugar if any more were added. The amount of sugar in one of these soft drinks equals the sugar content in seven average-sized apples. It's not uncommon for someone to drink three or four soft drinks per day, but can you imagine eating twenty-one to twenty-eight apples in one day?

Evidence is compelling: a steady diet of quick-fix convenience foods can take a toll on your mental wellness. And perhaps if we remove candy bars from the diets of violent people, they will become less aggressive. Dietary solutions for depression can be effective in the long term and certainly have fewer side effects.

7

Defending the Castle

OVER THE LAST TWENTY YEARS, a staggering amount of scientific discovery has clearly shown that food choices can either provide significant protection or be a significant risk for the nervous system. There is compelling evidence that certain foods and substances can protect against the major nervous system disorders. The food choices you make can help you defeat nervous system disorders that develop in adults, like Parkinson's disease and Alzheimer's disease. The research clearly suggests that inadequate diets and environmental factors play the starring roles in tragic brain disorders.

Chemotherapy, Memory Loss, and Cognitive Decline

Chemotherapy uses highly toxic agents to treat cancer; unfortunately, these agents also assault cognitive functions. Cancer patients who receive chemotherapy have displayed significant cognitive declines. Many women who receive chemotherapy report memory losses and an inability to concentrate. People receiving chemotherapy so commonly show memory loss that the medical community now calls this negative side effect of treatment "chemo-fog" or "chemo-brain."

Researchers have studied chemo-fog but found complex brain functions harder to measure than chemotherapy's physical side effects of nausea and lack of energy. However, critical studies that have been done have shown dramatic memory problems and language difficulties in people who received chemotherapy compared with cancer-free control groups. People who complete chemotherapy have lasting mental, language, and motor skill problems that continue well beyond their treatment periods. About half of the women actively receiving chemotherapy or who had recently finished a course of chemotherapy showed loss of cognition and memory declines. One study showed lingering mental problems up to two years after high-dose chemotherapy. (The study took into account the differences in educational levels, moods, and age.)

Most cancer patients experience some type of cognitive dysfunction. Cognitive decline may originate from the cancer disease process, but it also arises from the use of neurotoxic cancer treatments such as chemotherapy, immunotherapy, and radiation therapy.

More than 50 percent of immunotherapy patients who receive cytokines, items that up-regulate the immune system, display cognitive decline. For example, interferon therapy causes toxicity to the brain and nervous system problems such as emotional and psychiatric problems, lethargy, and confusion.

If you find yourself confronted with a cancer diagnosis and need chemotherapy or other treatments, you may use the dietary and lifestyle suggestions outlined in this book to lessen the neurotoxicity of the cancer treatments.

Bypass Surgery and Mental Deterioration

Every year over a half a million people in the United States undergo a heart bypass operation. While advances in surgical techniques and anesthesia have made the procedure safer, the risk of cognitive decline has not decreased.

Recent studies have confirmed the high incidence and persistence of cognitive decline in patients following bypass operations. Studies show that up to 75 percent of heart bypass patients demonstrate significant cognitive decline after their surgery. These patients displayed reduced cognitive function immediately after surgery and will likely suffer the effects permanently. Some mental impairments lasted at least five years after bypass surgery. Anesthesia caused temporary mental impairment, but did not cause the lasting cognitive decline.

Cardiologists are well aware that heart bypass operations cause mental deterioration, although they have not yet agreed about the precise mechanism causing the mental decline. Heart bypass operations create many brain-hostile conditions such as a lack of oxygen, inflammation, and amnesia-causing anesthesia drugs. During surgery, tiny blood clots shower the brain from the bypass pump that circulates and oxygenates the blood during the operation when the heart is stopped.

Three different steps of the procedure form blood clots that can impact the brain: 1) clamping and unclamping the aorta (a large vessel leading from the heart) loosens and frees plaques into the blood moving toward the brain; 2) the use of the bypass pump generates tiny blood clots; and 3) the attachment of the bypass vessel to the aorta can also break loose fatty plaques into the bloodstream that then make their way to the brain.

All bypass operations clamp off the aorta or large blood vessel at the top of the heart. The clamping disrupts and loosens the plaque deposits on the inside of this large vessel. At the end of the operation, when the clamp is removed, the loosened deposits shower the vessel with small blood clots, or micro-emboli, that eventually reach the brain. The tiny clots that reach the brain stop the blood flow in critical areas and cause a number of mini-strokes. The severity of the mental impairment that results relates directly to the amount of blood vessel blockage in the brain.

If you must have a heart bypass operation and you want to protect your brain, first, change your diet. A little-known option that very few cardiologists share with their patients is Dr. Dean Ornish's clinically and scientifically proven diet program that reverses heart disease. I encourage anyone grappling with the difficult prospect of having a bypass operation to contact Dr. Ornish and try his clinically proven dietary program to reverse heart disease (*Dean Ornish's Program for Reversing Heart Disease*, Random House, 1990).

Diet and Medications Can Damage Sensory Organs

Medications and Hearing Loss

Over a lifetime, noisy work and urban environments can lead to permanent hearing loss. Well-known causes of permanent hearing loss include loud noises or acoustic trauma. The incidence of hearing loss in the industrialized countries normally increases dramatically with advancing age. Yet more young people have hearing loss now than ever before. One study that evaluated the hearing abilities of incoming college freshman revealed that 60 percent had measurable hearing loss and 14 percent had hearing loss equivalent to that of an average sixty-five-year-old.

But noise is not the only cause of hearing loss. Modern-day hearing loss in developed countries can result from cumulative exposure to noise as well as from drug toxicity and environmental factors such as pollutants. A study conducted on a Sudanese tribe living in the African bush, far from urban development, discovered that people of this tribe at any age had better hearing when compared with a group of American farmers. The older members of the Sudanese could hear as well as the younger members. These people did not have exposure to urban work noises and drugs that harmed their hearing.

Many people don't realize that many toxic drugs also harm their hearing and can cause irreversible hearing loss. The medications include common drugs like aspirin and antibiotics like neomycin. Common aspirin causes hearing loss, particularly at high doses. In fact, studies show that aspirin use and exposure to noisy environments have a greater collective effect on hearing loss than exposure to only one of these hearing loss risk factors.

Diuretics such as Lasix, often used in the treatment of heart ailments, also affect hearing. Many of the toxic drugs used in chemotherapy cause hearing loss. Women treated for breast cancers often report hearing loss. Some popular antibiotics like erythromycin or amoxicillin can produce hearing loss in vulnerable people. But some of the most potent antibiotics from the aminoglycoside family, including amikacin, gentamicin, kanamycin, netilmicin, paromomycin, and tobramycin, can cause permanent hearing loss. Older people with fragile immune systems typically receive these powerful aminoglycoside antibiotics before or after surgery to prevent infection. Neomycin, an active ingredient in triple antibiotic ointments, is used to prevent infection from cuts, abrasions, and burns on the skin.

A hearing-friendly antiseptic, hydrogen peroxide offers a cheaper alternative to antibiotic ointments.

Dairy Products and Cataracts

Cataracts, one of the leading causes of blindness, are opaque areas that develop gradually within the lens of the eye and decrease vision. Cataracts result when the lens proteins degrade and lose their transparency. The example of egg whites turning opaque after cooking is often used to describe the process whereby less light passes through the affected lens of the eye.

Cataracts have been linked to eating dairy products. An expanding body of evidence shows that people who regularly drink milk have a greater number of cataracts compared with those who rarely consumed dairy products.

Specifically, a number of sugars contained in dairy products likely cause

Risk Factors for Cataracts

—High intake of dairy products

—Smoking

—Diabetes (especially if untreated)

—Long-term exposure to ultraviolet light

—Poor nutrition (especially a diet lacking plants)

—Medications (especially antibiotics, aspirin, antihistamines, and steroids)

—Excessive alcohol intake

Tips for Preventing Cataracts

—Consume diets that are high in antioxidants. Foods that provide good sources of antioxidants include nuts such as walnuts and seeds such as pumpkin seeds; blueberries; citrus fruits; strawberries; and dark green, yellow, orange, and red vegetables and fruit.

—Take supplements if your diet is not rich in antioxidants. Good anticataract supplements include vitamins C and E, beta-carotene, lycopene, lutein, and selenium.

—Avoid smoking. If you are a smoker, make sure you take antioxidant supplements, especially vitamins C and E.

—Avoid highly refined and hydrogenated oils and the foods that contain them.

—Use eye protection such as wraparound sunglasses that completely shield the eye, and always wear a hat in direct sunlight.

cataracts. Galactose, a sugar derived from the milk sugar lactose, degrades the proteins of the lens, thus causing cataracts. The sugars galactose and lactose are often referred to as "cataractogenic sugars." Studies conducted as long ago as 1935 have shown that lactose produced cataracts in rats. In humans, high blood levels of galactose have been linked to the formation of cataracts. The galactose found in dairy products, especially in yogurt, has also been linked to ovarian cancer.

Defending the Castle Against Nervous System Disease

An impressive amount of scientific information clearly shows that certain compounds in food can provide significant protection from cancer, heart disease, and brain disorders. For years most people believed that growing old normally brought a course of diseases such as Parkinson's disease, Alzheimer's disease, and senile dementia. However, research has shown that we don't have to sit back and wait to become helpless victims of brain disease.

But with the good news comes the bad—that we knowingly or unknowingly bring cognitive decline upon ourselves. The foods you eat can either prevent or nourish brain disease.

Parkinson's Disease

Researchers have struggled for more than a century to figure out what causes Parkinson's disease. Mystery solved: foreign chemicals such as pesticides have been shown to cause this devastating disease.

The symptoms of Parkinson's, like most diseases, vary from individual to individual. Some patients may notice malaise or an increase in sleepiness. Others notice an increase in shakiness or hand tremors, a decrease in voice projection, or handwriting that becomes cramped and spidery. Individuals may experience loss of thought or word patterns and feel depressed for no apparent reason. Friends and family members may notice the masked-face appearance of afflicted individuals, a face that lacks animation or expression. They may also notice the stiff, unsteady gait and slow movement of the individual. In some afflicted individuals, the disease does not progress quickly; however, in others the disease may cause severe motor disability in a dramatically short period.

The brain messenger dopamine helps to complete a circuit that coordinates the normal movement of muscles. When large decreases in dopamine cells occur (80 percent or more), the nerve cells fail to move the muscles properly. which results in jerky, unsteady actions. Drops in dopamine levels result in the typical shaking and tremors associated with Parkinson's disease.

Risk Factors for Parkinson's Disease

—Animal products, especially red meat
—Organ meats, especially kidney
—Low intake of fresh fruit and vegetables
—Living in an industrialized country
—Industry; living near a paper mill
—Occupation as farmer or pesticide worker
—Rural drinking water (well-water)
—Heavy metals, such as iron, manganese, and aluminum

Environmental Chemicals in Food and Well-Water Are Linked to Parkinson's Disease

Studies have shown a correlation between incidences of Parkinson's disease and industrialization, pesticide exposure, and consumption of water from wells. Heavy metals, such as iron, mercury, manganese, and aluminum—all byproducts of industry—have been shown to increase the risk of Parkinson's. These studies support efforts to address environmental causes to reduce the incidence of Parkinson's.

Iron accumulation in dopamine-producing areas of the brain has been found to cause nerve cell loss. Aluminum does not promote lipid (fat) peroxidation, but greatly increases the ability of iron to promote fat breakdown. Aluminum easily crosses through the stomach because of the high acidity of the digestive fluids in the stomach. The metal manganese also causes a Parkinson-like disease.

Drug-induced Parkinson's has resulted from use of a variety of drugs, both illegal and legal. Many believe drugs prescribed for psychiatric disorders, such as chlorpromazine and haloperidol, cause Parkinson's symptoms. Drugs such as metoclopramide for stomach disorders and reserpine for high blood pressure may also cause Parkinson's.

Cases of plant-induced Parkinson's disease found on the island of Guam during World War II may have resulted from the consumption of cycad plant flour during wartime shortages of staple foods. Parkinson's has been caused by a number of chemicals including carbon disulfide, carbon monoxide, the synthetic heroin contaminant MPTP, and paraquat. Many pesticides like paraquat released into the environment have structures very similar to that of MPTP. The higher incidence of Parkinson's in rural farming areas and areas that get most of their water supply from wells correlates with the increased use of pesticides in these areas.

People who drink well-water in agricultural areas whose water supplies are contaminated with multiple pesticides have a much higher risk for Parkinson's. Studies conducted in Madrid, Spain, also identified an increased risk of Parkinson's in people drinking well-water for more than forty years.

Other studies showing the agricultural influences on Parkinson's have been conducted in the United States and Canada. One agricultural area south of Montreal uses pesticides intensely, sells more L-dopa (used to treat Parkinson's), and has a higher mortality rate from Parkinson's disease than other metropolitan locations.

Diet and Prevention

What precautions can you take to prevent Parkinson's?

- Decrease your exposure to paraquat and other similar pesticides by eliminating from your diet crops that utilize paraquat, like plantation crops and citrus crops. Your best bet is to buy all organic fruits and vegetables.
- Avoid nondairy creamers, baking soda, baking powder, and commercially prepared baked goods. Aluminum is widely used in

these products as an anticaking agent. You can find nonaluminum baking soda in natural food stores.

- Avoid eating red meats and organ meats. Cadmium, a dangerous heavy metal, is commonly found in organ meats.

Alzheimer's Disease

Alzheimer's disease (AD) has been called the disease of the century. It has no known cure, and the disease is on the rise. A large portion of the aging baby-boomer population now shows typical signs of AD. The estimated number of patients in the United States with this debilitating brain disorder will almost quadruple in the next fifty years from four to fourteen million afflicted. About 360,000 new cases occur per year, equaling 980 new cases per day or 40 new cases every hour.

Each year, four million Americans will suffer from AD, the leading cause of dementia among people over the age of sixty-five. People with AD will experience a progressive loss of mental functions including memory, learning, attention, and judgment. The disease eventually leads to death. The crippling disease affects older Americans: 10 percent of people over sixty-five suffer from the disease. In those who reach eighty-five, which happens to be the fastest-growing age group in America, one-half will suffer from the debilitating effects of AD.

Two common neurological changes take place in the brains of people with AD. Alzheimer's patients suffer from a progressive loss of cognitive function due to a buildup of amyloid beta-containing plaques in the brain and the formation of neurofibrillary tangles in the nerve cells.

Alzheimer's disease usually begins in the sixth decade of life. The condition typically results in progressive impairments in memory, cognition (planning, insight, judgment), motor function, language, and visual and spatial perception. Apathy, commonly found in the initial stages, often turns to agitation as the disease progresses. Depression typically occurs in about half of diagnosed patients. Delusions, focal difficulties, seizures, and gait changes may also occur.

The disease eventually kills nerve cells in the basal forebrain, hippocampus, and cerebral cortex. Vital to memory, the hippocampus consolidates memories by controlling different parts of brain that together make up a complete memory and it decides which memories to preserve for the long term or to delete, as in short-term memory.

Three main features typify AD: plaques, neurofibrillary tangles, and reduced production of acetylcholine (an important brain messenger) in the hippocampus.

Risk Factors

Age, genetic factors, pollutants, pesticides, and heart disease are the most significant risk factors for the onset of AD. Risk factors associated with heart disease also increase the risk of AD. In a recent study, heart disease and high blood pressure increased the risk and prevalence of AD, where the risk multiplies in frequency and severity with advancing age. Other risks (smoking, alcohol consumption, and diabetes) most likely contribute to less severe brain impairments.

Cholesterol. A harmful cascade of events occurs when a person's blood cholesterol levels remain at high levels. Excess blood cholesterol causes metabolic change, including increased formation of free radicals that harm the integrity of the BrainGate. Through a complicated series of reactions, the cell membrane making up the BrainGate is damaged, cellular dysfunction ensues, and, if enough cell damage occurs, cell death may result. High blood cholesterol may result in a harmful event that causes a leaky BrainGate, allowing more toxic items to cross it.

Risk Factors for Alzheimer's Disease

—Brain injury (trauma)
—Pesticide exposure (carbamates, organophosphates, and chlorinated compounds)
—Heavy metal exposure (cadmium, lead, mercury, aluminum)
—Heart disease
—High blood pressure
—Age (increased risk at greater age)
—Gender (females have increased incidence)

High Blood Pressure. A fairly immediate result of high cholesterol is high blood pressure or hypertension. As cholesterol builds in the vascular system, blood pressure elevates, creating hypertension. Hypertension is a well-known risk factor for AD. As we age, the BrainGate normally becomes a bit weaker. This weakness, combined with the increased force of the high blood pressure, allows more proteins and other items such as toxic pollutants to slip past the BrainGate. Over time, increases in such breaches of the BrainGate may start the complex steps leading to AD.

Aluminum. Aluminum is a known neurotoxic agent linked to AD. Aluminum exposure can come from a number of sources, including the use of aluminum cooking vessels to prepare acidic foods that leach the aluminum into them. Researchers have shown that aluminum can cross the BrainGate and cause nerve cell death.

Silica-rich foods such as carrots block the uptake of aluminum from the gut. People exposed to aluminum in drinking water showed a dramatic decrease in the uptake of aluminum when they also received silica.

Once aluminum crosses into the brain, it causes multiple toxic actions such as the disruption of calcium control. The brain uses controlled changes in calcium levels to transfer signals required for proper brain communication.

Persons with AD also have increased tissue and blood levels of aluminum. Although researchers do not fully agree over the exact location and mechanism of aluminum buildup, some elderly people have brain levels over 20 times higher than those of a middle-aged group.

Mercury. Mercury has also been connected to AD. One study found that blood mercury levels in patients with AD were more than twofold higher than in people without AD.

Fish and shellfish contain mercury (methylmercury), and mercury vapors have been demonstrated to cross the BrainGate. Methylmercury is fat-soluble, which allows it to cross the BrainGate easily. Methylmercury can also bind to the amino acid cysteine and form a complex that resembles another amino acid called methionine. Studies in animals showed enhanced brain uptake of methylmercury when they were also given cysteine. The brain actively transports methionine, and the mercury–cysteine complex can piggyback across by this pathway, since its chemical structure mimics methionine.

Once mercury crosses the Brain-Gate, a number of toxic processes occur. Mercury creates an oxidative stress by depleting antioxidants. This depletion then blocks the formation of the brain messenger acetylcholine. The decrease in acetylcholine occurs mostly in the brain cortex and hippocampus.

Lead. Studies have revealed dramatic correlations of early toxic lead exposures that in later years caused over threefold greater risks for developing AD. Lead inhibits formation of the white fatty sheath called myelin that surrounds and protects nerve fibers. Another study looked at people with AD and vascular dementia and also found altered fats in the myelin sheath, a typical target of toxicity.

Seafood Sources of Mercury

Fish that tend to have high levels of mercury are usually predators and have sharp teeth

—Tilefish
—Swordfish
—King mackerel
—Shark
—Tuna (fresh, frozen, or canned)

Fish that generally have low levels of mercury

—Salmon
—Shrimp

Pesticides. Pesticide exposure is yet another risk factor for AD. Human studies show a higher prevalence of AD in rural farming environments where pesticides are used intensively. Pesticides can cross the BrainGate, form free radicals, cause oxidative stress, cause nerve cell death, and inhibit acetylcholine and energy production. These toxic effects parallel those observed in AD and other brain diseases such as dementia and Parkinson's disease.

Diet and Prevention

Alzheimer's disease is a very complex disease that likely results from a combination of factors that interact to create conditions that favor its development. What can you do to help your body avoid setting the stage for Alzheimer's? Eating a plant-based diet will lower your intake of cholesterol. Animal products contain high amounts of cholesterol that not only cause heart disease, but perhaps contribute to AD as well.

Dietary aluminum must also be minimized by avoiding high aluminum-containing antacids such as Mylanta, Remegel, and Rolaids. A diet high in whole, fresh vegetables and fruits will provide protection from the uptake of aluminum. Silica from plants prevents the absorption of aluminum from the gut.

A recent study showed that high intake of antioxidant vitamin C, vitamin E, and flavonoids will also lower the risk of AD. These antioxidants might decrease the risk of AD by reducing the oxidative stress in the brain and also by protecting against DNA damage and nerve cell death. These antioxidant vitamins may help treat existing mild to moderate stages of AD. It has been demonstrated that vitamin E slows the progress of AD by protecting brain cells. Because AD and heart disease go together, a diet rich in antioxidants should also decrease the risk of AD by lowering the risk of heart disease. In addition to antioxidants, other dietary nutrients protect against AD.

Dietary Components to Enhance Nervous System Function and Prevent Alzheimer's

Dietary Component	Sources
Vitamin E	Grains, nuts
Vitamin C	Citrus fruits, kiwi, sprouts, broccoli, cabbage
Magnesium	Supplements, spinach, melon
Flavonoids	Blueberries, green tea, red wine
Folic acid	Supplements
Methionine	Supplements
Ginkgo biloba	Supplements

Magnesium. Over three hundred different enzymes in the human body require magnesium and many of these are crucial to brain function. For example, magnesium assists the enzymes that convert waste ammonia for removal. If ammonia levels rise enough they can decrease your ability to think and concentrate. Magnesium maintains the electrical activity of nerve cells and helps convert dietary fatty acids into the brain-critical fat DHA. Deficiencies in essential fats like DHA have been associated with Alzheimer's disease.

Magnesium participates in building the protective myelin sheath that insulates the nerve fibers and activates almost all the key enzymes needed to produce and store energy. Poor magnesium intake is due to the limited amounts found in the typical high-fat, overprocessed, and overcooked American diet. Stress, caffeine, and alcohol consumption can also accelerate magnesium loss.

Folic Acid. Human studies show that low intake of folic acid is a risk factor for AD. Food sources for folic acid include those listed on page 100.

Ginkgo Biloba. Ginkgo extracts from the leaf of the ginkgo biloba tree are among the most common natural treatments for memory decline. Ginkgo extracts increase blood flow to the brain and have antioxidant properties, although the exact protective mechanism is unknown.

In Europe, people use extracts of ginkgo biloba to treat symptoms associated with cognitive disorders. In one study, about 37 percent of the AD patients tested showed improvement when given ginkgo biloba, and the study concluded that ginkgo biloba was both safe and able to stabilize and improve cognitive performance.

Some controversy still exists over whether ginkgo extract provides true mental protection, since some studies have not shown this result. However, in one yearlong study, subjects with dementia and AD given ginkgo showed stabilized or improved mental functioning and social interactions. Ginkgo also proved safe for use during the study, and researchers suggested that it may also prevent or delay further mental declines.

The scientific evidence suggests that you can reduce the risk of AD by changing dietary and lifestyle factors, especially by adopting those that promote a healthy heart. A high dietary intake of antioxidants and a significantly reduced dietary exposure to heavy metals and pesticides are two good ways to start.

Senile Dementia

Since the brain is a hungry organ requiring a rich supply of glucose and oxygen to function properly, it makes sense that anything that maintains a proper blood supply to the brain will also keep cognitive function at an optimal level. Many non-Alzheimer's forms of dementia result from a poorly functioning circulatory system, known as vascular dementia. People with advanced vessel and heart disease do not receive an adequate blood supply to the brain; thus mental decline ensues. In addition, many of these people also may suffer from a number of strokes that dramatically affect brain functions.

Diet and Prevention

You can help control vascular dementia by maintaining blood pressure, cholesterol, and fats (triglycerides) in the normal range. Eating a plant-based diet can help you lower most risk factors by bringing blood pressure, cholesterol, and fats back down to healthy levels. Changing certain lifestyle factors—like obesity, cigarette smoking, and lack of exercise—will also help you reduce your risk of vascular dementia.

o

Anti-Vascular Dementia General Meal Plan

Dietary Element	**Sources**
Antioxidants	Vitamins A, C, and E; beta-carotene; flavonoids
B vitamins	Vitamins B12 and B6, folic acid, biotin, niacin
Trace minerals	Selenium, copper, zinc, magnesium, manganese (Use the RDA for guidelines for vitamin intake. Most of the vitamins and minerals can be found in a quality multivitamin.)
Foods	Fresh fruit and vegetables. Red wine; dark grapes; green tea (high in antioxidants and manganese); garlic; high-fiber foods; chocolate; flavonoids; mono-unsaturated fats (olive and sesame oils); DHA supplements (Neuromins); brazil nuts, almonds, pecans, and walnuts
Miscellaneous	Aspirin (one every other day and use enteric-coated version)

Avoid High-fat diets; animal products (dairy products, poultry, meats); high-iron-content foods like red meat; trans-fatty acids, found in margarine and other products that include partially hydrogenated vegetable oils; fried foods, since they contain oxidized fats and cholesterol.

Part III

The Neuroenhancing Lifestyle

The 6-Step Brain-Purifying Program

YOU HAVE A BASELINE mental acuity at any given time. Here's how to optimize it! In the following pages you'll find an easy-to-follow detoxification and nutrition program to jump-start you on the way to better brain health by introducing new, brain-boosting items. You'll also find mental and physical exercises to reduce stress, and other lifestyle factors that can affect optimal brain functions.

We know that consuming more fresh fruits and vegetables and fewer processed foods and animal products offers one of the best ways to decrease your exposure to neurotoxic chemicals. Many persistent chemicals dissolve easily in fats and therefore concentrate in animal foods. These foods make up much of the American diet, including dairy products (especially cheese and ice cream), fish, meats, and foods processed with animal products.

The amount of time pollutants reside in your system, called the *half-life*, is the time needed for the body to get rid of half of the amount of pollutant stored in the body. Half-lives can range from minutes to years.

- The half-life of mercury is seventy days, but in the brain, it's 230 days.
- The half-life of cadmium is unknown, but may be as long as thirty years.
- The half-life of lead is more than twenty years.
- The half-life of dioxin is five to seven years.

Depending on the length of the half-life alone, some pollutant chemicals can stay in our bodies from cradle to grave. In fact, many toxic chemicals are transferred before birth from the pregnant mother to the fetus.

People are also exposed regularly to a wide variety of household and environmental chemicals, in the water they drink and the air they breathe. Many of these chemicals, such as lead, mercury, polychlorinated biphenyls (PCBs), dioxin, pesticides, and solvents are known neurotoxicants.

Step 1. Avoid or Limit Consumption of Neurotoxic Food, Drink, and Medication

Animal Products

Fat-filled meats (beef, pork, poultry, fish) and dairy products are responsible for over 95 percent of human exposures to dioxin and PCBs. Animal fats provide the largest exposure most people have to pesticides, antibiotics, and pollutants. To seriously reduce your exposure to toxic agents, you must lower your intake of animal products by limiting or eliminating red meat, dairy, and fish in your diet.

The chemical trichloroethylene (TCE) is used to degrease metal parts and in the manufacture of pesticides, adhesives, lubricants, paints, varnishes, and paint strippers. However, because of its widespread use, this highly toxic substance has found its way into our food supply. When ingested, TCE causes short-term memory loss, poor concentration, and difficulty solving problems. Margarine and meat products contain the highest levels of TCE.

Tap Water

Lead was once used extensively in commercial plumbing products, and many older homes may still contain lead-soldered plumbing and faucets. Even today, some of the most expensive plumbing fixtures currently sold contain some lead. Make sure to run the water for short periods before you use it to protect yourself from toxic effects of lead plumbing. You can also avoid exposure by never using hot tap water for cooking purposes, since it will likely contain more heavy metals in solution. Rice and vegetables cooked in lead-contaminated tap water will absorb about 80 percent or more of the lead contained in the cooking water. Therefore, ideally you should use a home water filtration system to ensure water quality (see Appendix). Reverse osmosis is considered the gold standard and the most complete and most permanent solution for water filtration problems. A number of water filters can effectively filter the water in limited applications such as the kitchen water supply used for drinking and cooking.

The presence of toxic metals in drinking water causes a large risk to brain health. Some of the major players include lead, mercury, cadmium, and arsenic. Chlorine added as a disinfectant unfortunately forms toxic chemicals called trihalomethanes that may cause cancer and high blood pressure, and they certainly do not support brain health. Many pesticides that may harm the brain have been carried into groundwater by rain

Trichloroethylene Concentration in Common Foods

Food	TCE Concentration *(parts per billion)*
Fish	10–100
Chinese-style sauce	28
Quince jelly	40
Crabapple jelly	25
Grape jelly	20
Chocolate sauce	50
Dairy products	0.3–13
Meats	**12,000–22,000**
Oils and fats	0–19
Fresh bread	7
Margarine	**440–3,600**
Yellow cake mix	1.3
Yellow corn meal	2.7
Fudge brownie mix	2.4
Beverages *(canned fruit drink, light ale, instant coffee, tea, wine)*	0.02–60
Fruits and vegetables *(potatoes, apples, pears, tomatoes)*	1.7–5
Bleached flour	0.77

Source: Agency for Toxic Substances and Disease Registry, 1993.

and irrigation. Asbestos-cement pipes have released microscopic asbestos fibers into some municipal water systems and have been linked to increased gut cancers.

We know that infants and children have more elevated and serious health risks than adults when exposed to toxic agents. Many substances easily excluded by an adult's fully developed BrainGate can easily enter into the vulnerable brains of children. Growing children absorb higher concentrations of toxic agents from their food and environment into their still-developing bodies. In children, the BrainGate is not yet fully developed, so it cannot provide as effective a barrier as that of an adult. Infants and toddlers often crawl on the floor and place toys and other nonfood items into their mouths, which results in a still greater exposure to environmental dusts that may contain toxic lead.

Dietary Sources of the Environmental Pollutant Dioxin

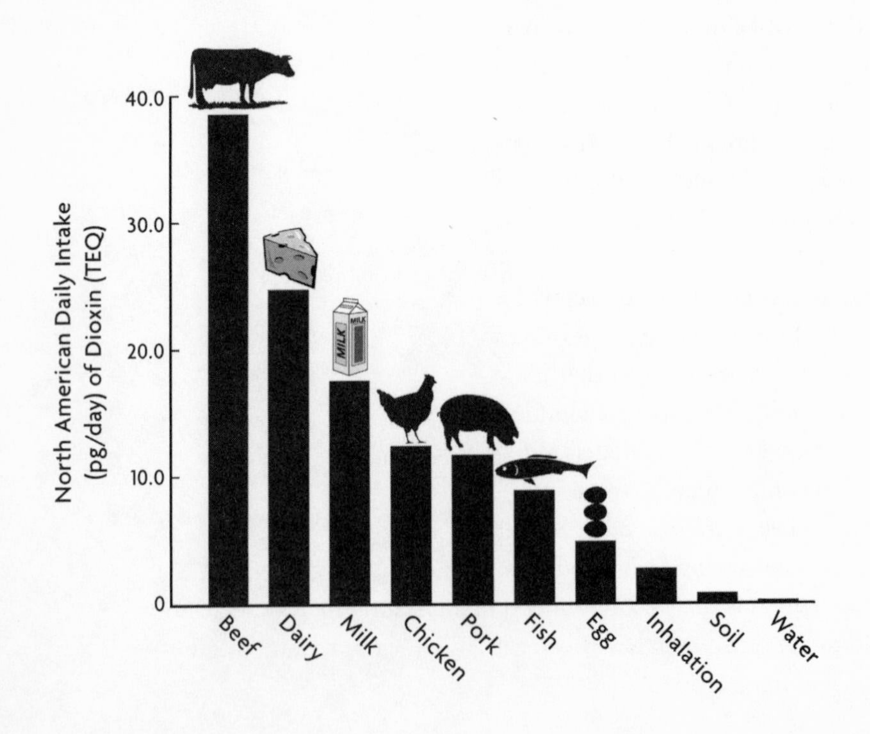

Lead harms the brain covertly: by the time its neurotoxic symptoms arise, irreversible brain damage has already been done. But there are things you can do to prevent or reduce your exposure to lead.

- Use a reverse-osmosis system to filter the water in your home.
- Drink only lead-free bottled or purified water.
- Check tap water for lead. Have an EPA-certified laboratory test your drinking water. If tap water has detectable lead, install a filtration system especially for water used in food preparation.
- Do not use ceramic dishes. Ceramic, pottery, or earthenware dishes may contain varying levels of lead. Do not serve food to children on such dishes unless you have determined they are lead-free.
- Do not use plastic mini-blinds.
- Avoid candle wicks that contain lead.
- Check soil lead levels. Check the lead levels and remove any contaminated soils from your child's play area. Soil abutting outside walls may have been contaminated from paint renovations.
- Test paint for lead. Test paint, dishes, and other substances with a lead kit.
- Keep children away from glossy, colored newsprint. Colored newsprint contains lead compounds and should not be burned in fireplaces.
- Use a high-efficiency particulate arrestor (HEPA) vacuum cleaner to remove small dust particles that conventional vacuums do not. HEPA filters have a 99.97 percent efficiency rating for removal of particulates 0.3 micron in size.
- Avoid exposure to cosmetics and dark hair dyes that contain lead.
- Limit the use of canned foods (especially imported), since they tend to contain high levels of lead.
- Avoid hobby materials that use lead. Avoid furniture refinishing, making stained-glass windows, indoor firing ranges (primer in bullets contains lead), pool-cue chalk (contains lead), and making lead-glazed pottery.
- Use lead-free calcium supplements.

- Consume a plant-based diet, since plant fiber is known to increase heavy metal removal. (Apples are particularly effective in this.)
- Increase dietary calcium, since calcium competes with lead for absorption. Eat high-calcium foods (see page 105).

Supplements and Antacids

Most consumers would cringe to discover that most major brands of calcium supplements and antacids contain significant levels of lead. Unfortunately, the manufacturing procedures for most supplements remain largely unregulated.

The lead testing of calcium supplements and antacids was sponsored by organizations such as the Natural Resources Defense Council, the Alliance to End Childhood Lead Poisoning, Physicians for Social Responsibility, and the Sierra Club. Dr. Russell Flegal conducted the analysis at the University of California Santa Cruz, Department of Environmental Toxicology.

The tables show the studies' reported lead values from the highest to the lowest levels.

Lead Levels in Antacids

Product Name	Calcium per Tablet *(milligrams)*	Lead Content *(micrograms)*
Di-Gel Advanced Formula Antacid (Schering-Plough Healthcare Products)	280 mg ($CaCO_3$)	0.4 to 4.6
Rolaids Antacid Tablets, Calcium Rich (Warner-Lambert Co.)	220 mg	0.4 to 4.5
Mylanta Soothing Lozenges Antacid, Calcium Rich Cherry Creme (Johnson & Johnson-Merck)	240 mg	0.1 to 1.5
Children's Mylanta Chewable Antacid, Fruit Punch and Bubble Gum Flavors (Johnson & Johnson-Merck)	160 mg	0.1 to 0.2
Children's Mylanta Liquid Antacid, Fruit Punch and Bubble Gum Flavors (Johnson & Johnson-Merck)	160 mg	0.03 to 0.2

o

Lead Levels in Calcium Supplements

Product Name	Calcium per Tablet *(milligrams)*	Lead Content* *(micrograms)*
Source Naturals Calcium Light	150 mg	16.6 to 20.7
GNC Food Source Certified Calcium from Oyster Shell (General Nutrition Corporation)	250 mg	5.4 to 5.4
Country Life Hypo-Allergenic Calcium, Magnesium, and Zinc	500 mg	2.5 to 5.0
GNC Dolomite 11 Grain (General Nutrition Corporation)	158 mg	1.2 to 5.0
Rainbow Light Everyday Calcium Systems	300 mg	4.9 to 4.9
TwinLab Calcium Rich Prenatal	325 mg	4.6 to 4.6
Longs Calcium and Magnesium (Leiner Health Products)	333 mg	1.4 to 4.1
Sav-On Calcium, Magnesium and Zinc (National Procurement & Logistics Company)	333 mg	3.7 to 3.7
Your Life Natural Calcium and Magnesium USP (Leiner Health Products)	333 mg	3.6 to 3.6
Schiff BoneBuilder with Calcium	333 mg	3.4 to 3.4
Os-Cal 500 High Potency Chewable Supplements (SmithKline Beecham)	500 mg	2.2 to 3.4
Jarrow Formulas Bone-Up Microcrystalline Hydroxyapatite	167 mg	0.5 to 3.0
Caltrate 600 1 D High Potency Calcium Supplement with Vitamin D (Lederle and American Cyanamid Company)	600 mg	1.4 to 2.9
Walgreens Calcium 600 USP (Leiner Health Products)	600 mg	1.4 to 2.9
Spring Valley High Potency Calcium 600 Supplement with Vitamin D (Perrigo Company)	600 mg	1.4 to 2.9
Solgar Calcium, Magnesium plus Boron (Solgar Laboratories)	333 mg	2.6 to 2.6
Your Life Natural Calcium, Magnesium and Zinc USP (Leiner Health Products)	333 mg	2.4 to 2.4
Nature Made 100% Oyster Shell Calcium 500 mg with Vitamin D (Pharmavite Corporation)	500 mg	1.9 to 1.9
Target Natural Oyster Shell Calcium (Distributed by Dayton Hudson Company)	500 mg	1.4 to 1.4
Posture-D High Potency Calcium with Vitamin D (Whitehall Laboratories, Inc.)	600 mg	0.2 to 0.5
Tums 500 Calcium Supplement, Chewable (SmithKline Beecham)	500 mg	0.3 to 0.4

** per minimum and maximum dose*

Step 2. Reduce Exposure to Toxic Chemicals and Containers in Your Kitchen and Household

Household Cleaners

Bon Ami is a great nontoxic cleaner, but you can also make simple, cleaning solutions with agents such as baking soda, soap, and vinegar. A vinegar solution provides an excellent cleaner for the scale or salt residues that water leaves after drying. The use of scrubbing pads and brushes can also eliminate the need for strong (and highly toxic) cleaning agents. The commercial household cleaning chemicals such as air fresheners, toilet deodorizers, disinfectants, and other cleaning solutions are known to contain solvents, some endocrine-disrupting chemicals, and, in some cases, even pesticides. Try less toxic or nontoxic cleaning products such as Seventh Generation (see Appendix).

Building Materials

Purchase nontoxic or less toxic alternatives when possible. Examples include solid wood furniture and natural-product carpets. Rather than carpeting wall-to-wall, select larger area rugs made from natural products that do not require formaldehyde-based adhesives for installation. Wood products such as plywood, chipboard, some types of carpeting, and even furniture can release volatile organic chemicals such as formaldehyde and other toxic compounds.

Installed carpets can serve as reservoirs for toxic pollutants, such as lead and pesticides, and need frequent vacuuming with a rotary brush and HEPA vacuum (see Appendix). Family members should remove their shoes when entering the house, since shoes can contaminate the household with lead and pesticides.

Aluminum

Some convincing studies reveal that diseased brains from Alzheimer's patients contain two to three times more aluminum than people without Alzheimer's. However, other challenging studies have shown no elevated disease risk for people exposed to high levels of aluminum. While the debate continues as to whether aluminum causes Alzheimer's disease, you should probably use vigilance and reduce your aluminum intake. Aluminum is toxic to the brain and interrupts over fifty brain-chemical reactions.

So, regardless of whether aluminum ever emerges as the main cause for Alzheimer's, it's critical to proper brain health to restrict your intake and exposure to aluminum. For example, kidney dialysis patients exposed to aluminum-containing binding agents during dialysis exhibited increased mental impairment. In addition, animals that have been administered aluminum compounds directly into the brain have also shown cognitive declines.

Step 3. Follow the NeuroNutrition Brain-Purifying Diet

Start eating according to the principles of a brain-purifying diet, and you will actually remove pollutants from all areas of the body. Once you understand the source of toxins in your diet, it will be easier to follow the general strategies of the Brain-Purifying Diet.

Eliminating Aluminum Exposure

Avoid the Following Foods:

—Processed foods (especially cheeses, cookies, canned foods, packaged cereals, pancake mixes)

—Iodized table salt

—Gelatin (Jell-O)

—Nondairy creamers

—Baking soda, baking powder

—Baked goods, unless baked with non-aluminum baking sodas

—Dietary supplements that use aluminum as a binding agent

Fortify Your Body:

—Drink bottled water.

—Reduce uptake of aluminum by increasing your intake of calcium-rich foods.

—Increase silicon intake, since it reduces uptake and removal of aluminum. Dietary sources of silicon include unrefined grains, whole-grain cereal products, and fresh root vegetables such as carrots.

Around the House:

—Do not use aluminum cookware.

—Use only glass containers and stainless steel pots for cooking.

—Use nontoxic household cleaners.

—Remove all antacids (Mylanta, Rolaids, Remegel) and analgesic pain relievers (NSAIDS) from the medicine cabinet.

Eat Fresh, Whole, Naturally Occurring Foods

Limit, or do not consume, any canned foods and overprocessed foods that are depleted of neuropreventive agents in your diet. Limit or eliminate fish because mercury can deposit in the muscle of fish, not the fat. The predatory fish contain the highest amounts of mercury and include swordfish, shark, and freshwater fish like the bass and northern pike. Tuna contains moderately high levels of mercury, and intake should also be limited. High levels of mercury are found in shark, swordfish, walleye, sea bass, and largemouth bass as well.

Greatly reduce or eliminate your intake of animal products such as meat, seafood, and dairy products.

For the best protection, adhere to the brain-purifying diet all the time. If you have to change your diet, do so only on the weekends. To help your body rid itself of pollutants, be sure to drink plenty of purified water to increase chemical removal through urine.

Fiber. Fiber is important for helping your body rid itself of the toxins it encounters every day. Be sure to include at least some measure of fiber in your diet every day.

Toxin-Removing Fiber Foods

Fiber	Pollutants Removed
Wheat bran	Binds cadmium, mercury
Rice bran, spinach fibers	Binds PCBs
Oat bran, psyllium	Binds bile
Pectin (apples) and carrots, cabbage	Lead
Silica, silicon (in root crops like carrots)	Aluminum

Antioxidant/Energy Foods. Feast on fruits (especially blueberries and other dark-blue or purple fruits), green tea, antioxidant spices, tomatoes, carrots, and organic dark chocolate. Dark chocolate is a rich source of antioxidant flavonoids and has much less contamination from neurotoxic lead. It's important to use only organic chocolate: 70 percent of the world's chocolate originates from West Africa, where they still use leaded fuels that contaminate the cacao plants, which then transfer to the chocolate.

Essential Fats. We know that humans can make all but two of the various fats required for nutritional health called essential fats. The two exceptions are omega-3 and omega-6 fats. Nuts and seeds such as walnuts and flaxseeds are the best sources of essential fats. Fish that contain especially high amounts of DHA and EPA include salmon, herring, mackerel, sablefish, sardines, and tuna. Many believe salmon supplies a good source of omega-3 fats, but salmon raised in fish farms have much less omega-3 fats and contain antibiotic residues. And the omega-3 fats break down readily when salmon is subjected to high-temperature cooking. Limit or eliminate your intake of fish since cooking destroys essential fats and fish contains high levels of environmental pollutants such as mercury and PCBs.

Flaxseed oil, walnut oil, and soybean oil contain both essential fats. Organic, unroasted nuts or seeds such as walnuts and almonds are excellent sources of the essential fats. Walnuts and almonds can be added to salads or eaten as a snack. Flaxseed is an excellent oil for use in salad dressings. Olive oil is an excellent choice for omega-9 fat. Do not consume highly processed canola oil!

Organic Foods. Choose as many whole, fresh organic foods as you can. Select dark-colored fruits and vegetables such as blueberries, spinach, and broccoli. Organic foods not only have fewer brain-toxic residues than commercial produce, but for a number of reasons they also have a higher nutritional value.

NeuroNutrition Food Groups. Each general food group confers a unique nutrition that cannot be obtained by other foods. Therefore, just eating more fruits and vegetables will not provide complete brain nutrition. Instead, include members from each of the brain-enhancing food groups in your daily diet.

NeuroNutrition Food Groups

Onion group	Garlic, onions, asparagus
Cruciferous group	Broccoli, cabbage, cauliflower
Grass group	Corn, oats, rice, wheat (and whole-grain, unbleached flours)
Legume group	Soybeans, green and wax beans, peas
Solanace group	Tomatoes, potatoes
Umbelliferous group	Carrots and celery

Brain-Supporting Supplements. Take daily supplements from reputable companies (see Appendix). DHA, coenzyme Q10, and multiple vitamins provide especially important nutrition for older people. DHA helps build the foundation for brain health. Large doses of coenzyme Q10 may slow the progress of Parkinson's disease.

O

Brain-Supporting Supplements

Dietary Supplement	Recommended Daily Dose	Take with Meal
General		
Docosahexaneoic acid (DHA)	50–300 milligrams (Neuromins)	Yes
Coenzyme Q10	100–200 milligrams (Q-gel, 20–60 milligrams)	Yes
Multiple Vitamin and Minerals	Follow package instructions	Yes
Phosphatidylserine (PS) (Leci-PS)	100–300 milligrams	Yes
Acetyl-L-carnitine (ACL)	1–2 grams	No
N-acetyl-cysteine (NAC)	200–600 milligrams	No
Lipoic acid	50–200 milligrams	Yes
Choline	1–4 grams	Yes
S-Adenosylmethionine (SAM)	400–1200 milligrams	Yes
Pycnogenol	50–200 milligrams	Yes
Grape seed extract	50–200 milligrams	Yes
Ginkgo biloba extract	50–250 milligrams	Yes
B-family vitamins		
Vitamin B6	100 milligrams	Yes
Vitamin B12 (under the tongue)	100–1000 micrograms	Yes
Folic acid	400 micrograms	Yes
Antioxidant vitamins		
Beta-carotene	25,000 IU or 15 milligrams	Yes
Vitamin C (time release)	500–2000 milligrams	Yes
Vitamin E (mixed tocopherols)	400–1000 IU	Yes
Selenium	50–200 micrograms	Yes
If exposed to aluminum		
Silica	5–20 milligrams	Yes

Brain-Friendly Cooking

High-temperature cooking—deep-frying, grilling, and even microwaving—produces oxidized fats and other neurotoxic agents that weaken brain health. We know that eating a diet low in fat and sugar is healthy, but researchers have been puzzled by the fact that some people who eat this diet still become ill. To really eat healthy, you need to cook foods using lower-temperature methods such as steaming, broiling, boiling, light baking, and moderate microwaving, since these will preserve vitamins and omega-3 fats.

When preparing foods:

- Cook foods only in glass or stainless steel pots or dishes.
- Prepare foods using less fat and cooking oils. (Both plant and animal fats harm the gut in excess.)
- Replace corn oil with sesame oil for cooking.
- Replace butter with cold-pressed flaxseed oil.
- If you eat meat, choose only lean cuts and free-range varieties.
- Do not eat foods that show mold growth. Instead, freeze foods if not eaten within three to five days.
- Always use airtight food containers when refrigerating foods.
- Replace mayonnaise with Vegenaise® (see Appendix); it is available in four varieties: original, grapeseed oil, expeller-pressed, and organic. Other good choices for sandwich spreads are hummus, tahini, and mustard.

We know that eating excess refined sugar can increase the formation of toxic advanced glycation end products or AGEs. AGEs cause blood vessels to lose flexibility, leading to high pulse blood pressures that can harm the brain. Unfortunately, high-temperature cooking—deep-frying, grilling, and even microwaving some foods—can also form AGEs in the presence of high levels of sugars, fats, and proteins. AGEs form normally in the human body, but the more sugar, the more AGEs are created.

If you must prepare foods at high temperatures:

- Don't use red meat—it forms much higher mutagenic items when cooked at high temperatures.
- Coat foods with soy flour or cottonseed flour before cooking.
- Reduce heating times, to form fewer toxic agents.
- Before frying or charbroiling, briefly microwave the food and discard the cooking juices.
- Physically block foods from direct contact with flames, grilling surfaces, and charcoal.
- Use stainless-steel cooking sheets; do not use aluminum cooking materials.
- Do not eat the outer black charred areas of cooked foods, since that contains the greatest concentration of the most powerful toxic agents called mutagens.
- Avoid eating the skin of poultry.

To decrease the toxicity of foods cooked at high temperature:

- Eat more dietary fiber, since it helps reduce the toxic effect of high-temperature cooking. Fiber from corn and wheat bran lower the toxicity of charbroiled food when eaten together.
- Consume more fresh cruciferous vegetables when eating fried foods to reduce toxicity.
- Eat more omega-3 fats to decrease the toxicity of mutagens.
- Eat more dark-green leafy vegetables to reduce the toxicity of mutagens. Green tea may also decrease toxicity from cooking.
- Antioxidant vitamins A, C, E, and beta-carotene are also protective.

Brain-Friendly Cooking Oils. Only use cold-pressed oils (expeller) such as olive oil or sesame oil. Olive oil will burn at a lower temperature than sesame oil, but will still provide better nutrition than canola and corn, sunflower, or cottonseed oils. Macadamia nut oil, while difficult to find, is another good oil. Cold-pressed flaxseed oil can substitute for butter—use it on vegetables, popcorn, and corn on the cob. For cooking oils use only expeller or cold-pressed sesame, olive, or macadamia oil. Yet remember that high-temperature cooking destroys most of the essential fats and vitamin E in even the best oils.

Dining Out and Dining In—Brain-Friendly Choices

Whether you're on the road or staying in, you have many options for choosing healthy, brain-protective foods.

Restaurant Food. The restaurant business competes for each customer. How do they compete? The taste of their food has become their highest priority. How do most restaurants make food tasty? First, they use inexpensive hydrogenated fats, sugars, and salt in ingredients, and then they offer a rich selection of foods subjected to high-temperature cooking techniques such as deep-frying.

Therefore, on road trips, make sure to bring your own snacks and food to eat in order to limit restaurant stops. When in doubt, select salads and request the dressing on the side. Italian salad dressings usually contain brain-friendly olive oil. Or use lemon or lime juice in place of salad dressing.

Change Your Cuisine. Ethnic cuisines like Japanese, Italian, Indian, Thai, Mexican, Mediterranean, and Chinese offer many brain-protective foods. Ethnic foods often use olive oil, and meals tend to feature large amounts of steamed vegetables and brown rice, instead of meats. Request fiber-rich, less-processed brown rice instead of white rice if you can.

Italian and Mediterranean foods use olive oil and have pasta dishes that use generous amounts of garlic and onions. Japanese foods often use sesame oil, brown rice, and whole-grain noodles. Make sure to request MSG-free food in Asian restaurants.

Redefine Dessert. For desserts, explore soy ice creams, fresh fruits, Italian fruit gelatos, and frozen fruit bars. Organic Soy Delicious® is an excellent brand of soy ice cream (www.turtlemountain.com). Try fresh fruits. Most restaurants will offer mixed berries (add a little liquor like Grand Marnier) even if not listed on the menu. Once you remove dietary refined sugar, your taste threshold will readjust and fruit will taste very sweet! The complex and pleasurable tastes of fresh fruit will become apparent. High-sugar foods will taste sickeningly sweet—as they should!

Some great antioxidant fruits include cantaloupe, grapefruit, oranges, bananas, berries such as raspberries, strawberries, and blueberries, pears, and apples. Neuroprotective blueberries freeze very well, so you can have a brain-nourishing year-round supply. Use more low-sugar fruit spreads. Stay away from bleached, refined flour products; instead, select whole-grain cereals and breads, bagels, or oat bran pancakes.

Brainy Drinks. Blueberry smoothies blended from fresh blueberries, bananas, soymilk, and soy ice cream are delicious satisfying drinks. Fresh-squeezed orange juice has more antioxidant clout than the overprocessed, sugar-filled breakfast drinks. But don't overconsume fruit juices or you will propel your blood sugar levels out of balance and mental performance will suffer. It's better for the brain to eat whole oranges. Juicing fruits and vegetables degrades fibers and when you consume these drinks they cause a rapid increase in blood sugar, followed by low blood sugar that decreases brain energy.

Obtain quality green tea in bulk or loose form from oriental stores, since typical food stores carry low-quality tea. Sencha is an excellent green tea. To brew green tea, boil the water and allow it to cool to about 80 degrees C. Briskly boiling water destroys the protective polyphenols and makes the tea bitter. Adjust the amount of tea and brewing times according to your taste. While you may add sweeteners to green tea, do not add milk. Green tea also tastes great as iced tea.

Snacks. Eat more fruits: apples, oranges, peaches, grapes; and raw vegetables such as celery, carrots, and cucumbers. Purchase bags of prewashed and peeled baby organic carrots and other vegetables. Buy unroasted, unsalted almonds, walnuts, and pistachios.

Licorice is a great antioxidant snack. Panda-brand licorice from Finland uses real licorice root extract. Plain air-popped popcorn or popcorn cooked in a small amount of sesame oil provide good snacks. Use cold-pressed flaxseed oil in place of butter for topping. Remember that packaged microwave popcorn contains all the wrong things for your brain: it's loaded with hydrogenated oils and is high in fat and salt.

Soy. Decrease your intake of dairy by eating more soy products. An excellent soymilk is made by Silk (www.silkissoy.com). Silk makes an entire line of soy products, including coffee creamers and flavored soymilks. Soy products are available in a number of varieties. Tofu is formed from soymilk. Silken-type tofu can be used to make cheesecake, fruit smoothies, or anything with a creamy texture. You can grill regular tofu, or scrambled it like eggs for breakfast. Regular tofu comes in three forms: soft, firm, and extra firm, depending on your cooking needs.

- Use soymilk for coffee or black tea (not green tea).
- Use soymilk instead of regular milk in baked-goods recipes.
- Use soymilk in place of yogurt to make fruit smoothies.
- Add soy to Italian dishes and Oriental stir-fry dishes.
- Add tofu to chili, stews, and soups.

Step 4. Do Daily Mental Exercises to Enhance Brain Function

Keeping your brain young also involves mental exercises. The art of learning improves with time. Brain cells, just like muscle cells, need constant stimulation in order to maintain their healthy structure. The brain perpetually works by interacting with the world and collecting and processing stimuli, and then perceiving and finally acting on the collected information. A stimulating mental environment prevents cognitive decline just as much as physical activity does. Healthy people keep their brain young by constantly reading, learning, studying, staying curious, meeting new people, asking questions, and maintaining their excitement about this wonderful world.

You can learn new mental tasks and incorporate them into your day without taking additional time. For example, when you dress in the morning, try utilizing your nondominant hand to button your clothing and tie your shoes, brush your teeth, comb your hair, and shave. Start solving crossword puzzles as you read the newspaper.

Join a card-playing club and learn how to play bridge. Play verbally challenging games like Scrabble, or number-intensive games like Bingo, or strategy-focused games. Learn new skills like yoga, sculpture, salsa dancing, painting, or foreign languages, or join a computer club.

Stimulation Is Protection

Animal research shows that a stimulating environment actually protects the brain from some forms of toxic damage. For example, rats exposed to a stimulating mental environment were protected from some of the toxic and damaging effects of lead when compared with rats living in isolation. The degree that stimulating environments provided protection surprised the researchers. One can only imagine how these results would translate into brain health for the human populace.

A study tracked over five thousand humans ranging in age from twenty to ninety years. If the study participants displayed mental decline, they immediately completed five one-hour sessions designed to hone their mental skills. In 50 percent of the cases, the training sessions dramatically improved the subjects' mental functioning. Once again, the study revealed that a mentally stimulating environment preserves mental skills at any age.

The fear of losing his mind grated on the foreign news correspondent Terry Anderson while he was being held captive by Muslim extremists in Lebanon. Anderson was held captive for close to seven years in the mid-1980s. But Anderson practiced an acknowledged strategy of fighting mental decline by keeping his mind engaged. Anderson often pressed his fellow hostages into spirited political debates. He convinced a fellow captive to teach him a foreign language and created a unique form of sign language used to communicate among hostages. Learning new skills can prevent the loss of brainpower.

Maybe you've fallen into a routine life that does not require learning new skills. How can you incorporate new learning tasks into a typical day? Engaging in challenging conversation and reading new books are small yet significantly healthier tasks than passively watching TV.

To put your brain through serious mental paces requires you to learn a new language, play a musical instrument, sign up for college courses. Take up chess or some other complex game. Passively watching TV does little to engage your intelligence and flex higher brain skills. Studies continue to reinforce findings that people who engage in challenging intellectual pursuits do much better in retaining their cognitive abilities. Therefore, serious cognitive decline is not inevitable as we age. It's not unusual for an active person in her nineties to have sharp cognitive skills.

Traveling is yet another method for challenging your brain. For your next vacation, choose a non-Western country and immerse yourself in its culture, customs, cuisine, and language. Don't sign up for a group tour, though. Instead, plan your own trip and travel as a sensitive visitor, not just a tourist.

Many studies demonstrate that higher levels of education reduce the risk of contracting Alzheimer's disease. In one study, people who remained active both physically and mentally in their middle age contracted Alzheimer's disease three times less frequently. Researchers also found that people who engaged in less leisure activity between the ages of twenty and sixty years had a 3.85 times greater risk of developing Alzheimer's. Once again, mentally and physically inactive lifestyles do not foster healthy brains. Physical and mental activity allowed early humans to adapt to new environs by developing tools, farm implements, weapons, and the survival skills that they passed on to the next generation.

Exercises to Enhance Brain Function

—Travel to exotic countries
—Take computer classes
—Learn to play a musical instrument
—Start making home repairs and woodworking
—Learn how to paint or sculpture
—Become an avid reader
—Learn a new language
—Play more card games or board games
—Do the crossword puzzle in the daily paper

Protecting the Network

The brain is often described as having the quality of plasticity or adaptability. The brain can recruit new functional areas of the brain, which gives it a high degree of versatility. Your brain circuitry constantly reorganizes and restructures itself in response to the particular stimuli it receives and from new learning experiences. This complex interaction causes the brain's nerve fibers (dendrites) to branch and link to other nerve cells. The dendrites act like conduits in which nerve cells signal and communicate with one another. Robust, healthy neurons have the capacity to connect to thousands of other neurons. It's estimated that neurons can form well over a trillion different linkages—a network that forms the underlying foundations for the cognitive capacities of memory and thinking. The more we engage our brain in complex thoughts, the greater the degree to which nerve cells will branch and the sharper our brains will function independent of our age.

Inactivity can actually cause the loss of receptors in the nervous system. But if you become active again, you can gain back the use

The Brain Cell Network

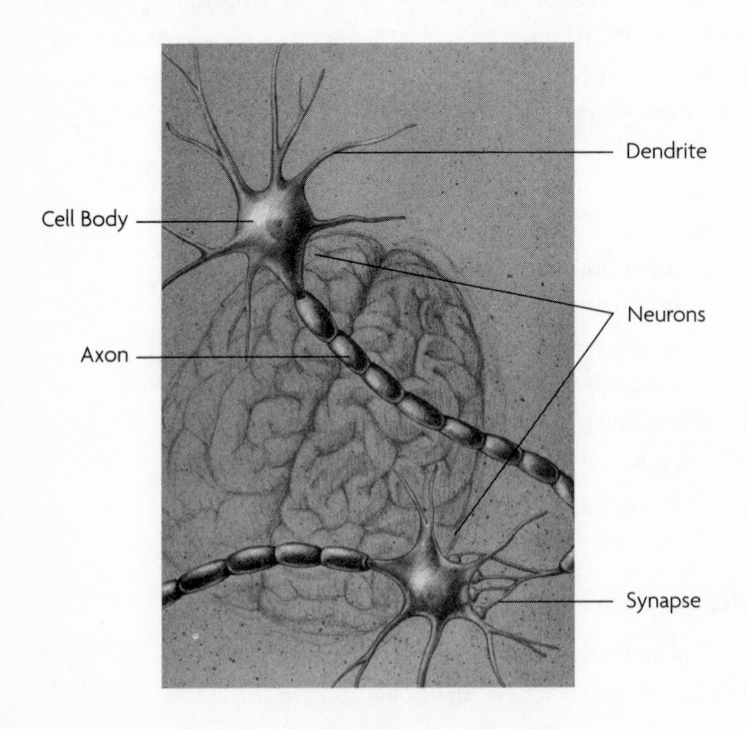

of those receptors. Most researchers think that the process of forming memory and learning results in changes at the nerve-to-nerve connection or synapse. The changes involve increases in receptor aggregation in the synapse. Research also shows that these synapse changes are required for the acquisition and storage of information. From the standpoint of survival, it appears that the plasticity of the brain to rework circuitry and its capacity to repair itself following injury use the very same methods that the brain uses to store memories. Therefore, since both memory formation and brain repair require a mentally stimulating environment, it's safe to conclude that cognitive skills and challenges become an integral component of preserving your memory over a lifetime.

Most people believe as you age you naturally lose significant quantities of brain cells and, therefore, lose cognitive function. But many studies have shown that age-related cognitive decline does not have to become an automatic consequence of old age. Researchers followed six thousand older people and gave them regular mental tasks over a ten-year period. About 70 percent of the people given stimulating mental tasks retained their cognitive powers with advancing age. This study supports the fact that older brains can still make and grow new neurons. Significant age-related cognitive decline usually results from an underlying disease such as heart or vascular disease. It's likely that in healthy older individuals, lack of stimulation for the brain or mental and physical inactivity causes most age-related mental declines.

Mental Exercises: Proven Strategies to Improve Memory

Mnemonics

Most people believe that a superior memory results from a high IQ, intellectual abilities, or more developed structures within the brain; however, a very recent study has shown that people with exceptional memories utilize special learning strategies and mnemonic techniques, not superior intellect or differences in brain structures. Mnemonics include memory strategies that assist in memory recall.

By employing particular mnemonic devices, researchers have even been able to improve memories in the elderly. In a recent study, people with superior memories mainly used a memory technique called the "method of loci." The method of loci, also called the "mental walk," is an ancient Greek mnemonic practice. It's believed to originate with the Greek poet Simonides in 477 B.C., who made use of very familiar locations or routes and visualizing objects and recalling them in order at key points along the route.

Put the method of loci into practice: Create a mental route by establishing a series of loci (places or locations) that you will use as a framework for later placing and memorizing objects. A locus can act as familiar things inside your home, such as paintings, a special wall, a microwave oven, a bathroom, bedroom, or dining room, or familiar buildings or structures along a well-known street.

1. First, chose a familiar place, such as outside on a well-known street with buildings, or inside your home.
2. Next, take a mental walk through a room in your house, visualizing each location in the room. Take note of the bookcases, color, shelving, furniture, and paintings.
3. Now construct a complete list of everything you wish to remember—say, six things you need for a romantic dinner: red wine, candles, tablecloth, flowers, chocolate, and music.
4. Link each item to a specific location in the room. For example, vividly visualize a bottle of red wine on the dining room table. Place the other five objects within other locations in the room.
5. Finally, take a mental walk and visually review each item in the location where you have put them. Later, when you need to recall your list, take the same mental walk and retrieve the various items in the order you placed them in the room.

The locations you chose to place items don't have to be brick-and-mortar buildings or any specific room. To remember what clothing to pack for a quick weekend trip, you can use your own body. Visualize your body carefully from head to toe and think of the clothing you will need for each body part or location. Start with a hat and sunglasses for your head, shirts, jackets, or skirts for your torso, and work all the way down to your toes. When you go to pack, use the same mental walk to recall the items you need. Use this mnemonic device for packing for frequent trips and you will rarely forget items for the trip.

Now, when you are confronted with a list of items or objects to commit to memory, you can visualize images for each of the items and place them in the loci or location along your mental route. To retrieve the items, you simply take a mental stroll through your house and ask yourself: What sits on the dining room table? What sits on the bookcase? and so forth, until you cover all the locations. When you link items with loci in your house, sometimes you will create ridiculous images. Yet the more silly or vivid the created image, the more easily you will recall it.

Mnemonic devices force you to think actively or to deep-process the information that ties it to material already stored in long-term memory. Mnemonic devices also provide an organizing framework that allows recall of one element that triggers the recall of the other elements. Most mnemonic devices use imagery, since it has the advantage of allowing the memorized material to become more vivid, concrete, and better recalled over time.

There are other forms of mnemonic devices besides the method of loci, of course: keyword and first-word mnemonics, acronyms, and rhymes or catchy phrases. All assist your memory, usually with imagery. Once again, the more vivid and funny the mnemonic images are, the easier the information is recalled.

Rhymes

Rhymes are an easy way to help you recall information. This popular rhyme helps many remember the number of days in a particular month:

Thirty days hath September,
April, June, and November;
All the rest have thirty-one,
Excepting February alone:
Which hath but twenty-eight, is fine,
'Til leap year gives it twenty-nine.

Rhymes aid memory, but can be hard to create for some material and are time-consuming.

First-Letter Mnemonics and Acronyms

First-letter mnemonics and acronyms use the first letter of each item or phrase that needs to be memorized to form an actual word. Each letter represents one component of the material to be memorized. Some common examples are: HOMES, to recall the names of the Great Lakes: *H*uron, *O*ntario, *M*ichigan, *E*rie, *S*uperior; and STAB, to recall the basic voices in a chorus: *s*oprano, *t*enor, *a*lto, and *b*ass.

To recall a person's name that you may have on the tip of your tongue, start reviewing the letters of the alphabet in order from A to Z and visualize the person at the same time you mentally recite the alphabet. Often recalling the first letter of the name is enough to access and recall the entire name.

Keyword Mnemonics

Keyword mnemonics are best suited for the recall of abstract and unfamiliar information and useful for learning a new language. For example, in the Japanese language, *tako* is the word for octopus in English. "Tako" sounds similar to "taco." So you can create a mental image of an *octopus taco* that is easily recalled from memory.

Step 5. Reduce Stress

Burned out?

Everyone—even the most blissful soul—has some sort of stress in daily life. But when does the intensity of stress become too much to handle? People claim that the most difficult type of stress arises when you have no control over its source, such as with externally imposed deadlines.

It's very difficult to quantify the level of stress in someone's life. Often the first indicator is a seemingly unwarranted angry outburst. A number of warning signs can help you recognize a stressful event:

- You lash out at people for little reason.
- You feel an unusual amount of anxiety and cannot concentrate.
- You feel unable to cope and are overwhelmed.
- You experience angry outbursts and have relationship stress.
- You have a continued sickness or illness.
- You become withdrawn and distant from friends.
- You suddenly don't seem to care about anything.
- You feel tired and fatigued most of the time.
- You suddenly become disorganized and forgetful.
- You physically let yourself go and don't maintain your personal hygiene.
- You drink more, or more heavily, than normal or abuse drugs.

How to Relax

When the workday becomes stressful and you feel the signs of burnout or you lash out at someone for little reason, stop for a moment and take a deep breath. Rather than respond quickly to a particularly stressful event, analyze the situation like a critical observer who needs to find humor from the episode.

You can manage stress by learning how to allow a healthy level of stress into your life, yet recognize the fact and take action when the level of stress becomes unmanageable. Everyone reacts to stress differently: learn how you react and develop appropriate techniques to reduce stress that best suit you.

Laugh. Laughter has been shown to release endorphins, the compounds that give marathoners that "runner's high." Alternatively, take a moment to think calm thoughts and visualize a tranquil setting. Or pop up from your desk and take a brisk walk around the block or up the stairs. If you can't do any of these things then take a series of slow, deep breaths. While not appropriate in many work situations, the act of crying naturally relieves stress. Emotional tears contain large amounts of stress-related substances like adrenaline.

Cultivate friends who enjoy telling jokes and who make you laugh. These types of friends can greatly reduce stress. A support network of friends also defuses stress. If you don't presently have a support system, get one. Don't forget that a personal support system can include pets as well.

In a seven-year study using seventy-year-old people, those with emotionally supportive networks showed better cognitive skills such as abstract reasoning, spatial ability, nonverbal and verbal memory, and language skills compared with those without such a network. In a five-year study of heart disease patients, those without spouses or close friends had a three times greater risk of dying than those with support groups.

Unplug the News. In today's information age, everyone becomes overwhelmed at some point by information overload. It's not surprising that too much information plagues us with a continued source of stress. If work remains increasingly stressful, unplug the daily news from your life. When the signs of stress surface, take a media/news fast. Drop your weekly newspaper subscription and keep only the Sunday paper. Don't watch the nightly news; instead, listen to a news radio or music station.

TV advertisements also can stress you out: use your mute button! Better yet, unplug your TV. Watch thought-provoking movies, videos, or DVDs instead. Don't let yourself become an expert on terrorism or politics; in today's world, obsessing on current affairs causes stress.

Simplify. Eliminate stress by simplifying your life—consolidate credit cards and bank accounts so you don't have to reconcile multiple accounts. Sign up for electronic payroll deposits and use automated payments for your utility bills. Buy only the same brand of socks in the same color so you can eliminate the need to match socks. This trick works especially well with white athletic socks that occupy one drawer in the dresser.

NO POSTAGE
NECESSARY
IF MAILED
IN THE
UNITED STATES

BUSINESS REPLY MAIL

FIRST-CLASS MAIL PERMIT NO. 551 WASHINGTON DC

POSTAGE WILL BE PAID BY ADDRESSEE

LifeLine Press
PO Box 97278
Washington, DC 20078-7350

Listen to Soothing Music. When you want excitement, play music with a fast rhythm. On the other hand, if you want to calm down, select music with a slower rhythm and let its gentleness relieve your stress.

Imagine. For a swift shift into a tranquil state of mind, use your imagination to transport yourself to calmer environs. In one study, a combination of music and guided imagery affected the moods and levels of the stress hormone cortisol. Healthy adults listened twice weekly to sessions of music and used guided imagery over a six-week period. The study participants reported significant reduction in depression and other mood disturbances, including fatigue. Even after the sessions, cortisol levels dropped significantly lower for up to six weeks.

Another study provides more evidence that image therapy may manage stress. People who listened to guided-imagery tapes for three days before and for six days following surgery displayed less pain and stress compared with a control group. Image therapy has also assisted sleep patterns and reduced stress in women suffering from post-traumatic stress disorder after sexual assaults. Other studies have investigated groups of highly stressed people by using stress-reducing yoga postures and techniques of meditation. The

Relaxation Techniques—Make Yourself Stressproof

—Adopt a positive,"can do" attitude.

—Begin an exercise routine (swimming, jogging, yoga, tai chi, weight training) and stick to it every day.

—Laugh out loud—find humor in stressful situations. Learn how to laugh at yourself.

—Remove yourself from the stressful environment and take a brisk walk.

—Start slow deep-breathing exercises and meditate.

—Take "power naps."

—Get professional massages.

—Post some supportive or inspirational quotes on your wall.

—Remove yourself from a noisy work environment. Go to an unused office or library or simply shut your office door and use earplugs.

—Use your imagination and visualize yourself on a peaceful beach or in another tranquil environment.

—Listen to calming music.

—Become introspective and philosophical—look at your stressful event as a learning experience and a challenge in life rather than a defeat.

—Develop excellent time management skills.

—Delegate tasks to others when your workload becomes too big.

—Nurture other coworkers and they will return the favor.

study reported a 54 percent average drop in psychological disorders compared with the control group.

Breathe. A powerful tool in your antistress arsenal is something many people overlook: conscious control of your breathing. Breathing, though an autonomic function, also remains under immediate voluntary control and if used properly can activate your relaxation response. When you first sense a stressful event, exhale completely and slowly inhale through the nose. Concentrate on expanding your diaphragm to assist in filling the lungs with air. Finally, make sure to expand your chest and perhaps even lift your arms to squeeze every last breath into your lungs. Then pause and slowly exhale the air from your mouth. Tighten your chest and stomach to completely remove any residual air. Pause briefly once more, allowing your body to relax, then start the cycle over until you feel the stressful feelings have passed. A number of stress clinics recommend similar breathing techniques to activate the relaxation response. Use breathing techniques as powerful ways to defuse stressful situations, since you always have this option.

Meditate. Meditation is another method to reduce stress. Deep-breathing exercises provide a good prelude to meditation. Listen to the sounds that emerge from deep breathing. Let your mind wander, daydream. Studies have found that meditation lowers the heart rate and blood pressure, and it's not surprising that it also lowers the stress hormone cortisol.

Utilize Aromatherapy. Another area gaining more recent acceptance is aromatherapy. Certain common smells or fragrances can transport you to the distant past. Pleasurable fragrances often have positive effects on emotional well-being. Studies show that citrus fragrances can reduce the need for antidepression medications, and lavender oil has a calming effect. So after a stressful day, draw a hot bath and add some of the essential oils like lavender oil.

Exercise. Recall the flight-or-fight response to stress, as covered in Chapter 4. This well-known stress response often leaves you with excess stress hormones circulating in the blood. Use vigorous exercise to purge your body of these hormones. Hit the gym. Punch a punching bag, or go for a run or a bike ride. After all, the flight-or-fight response prepares you to react physically to pending danger. If you can't leave the office right then, close your office door and do a few jumping jacks. Do some push-ups or sit-ups, or take a walk up and down some stairs or around the block. At the end of the day, do some yoga stretches or tai chi movements.

Extremely stressful situations increase a person's vulnerability to illness and disease. Researchers discovered that people who stick to a regular exercise program are much less likely to become ill after experiencing stressful events. Further, in animals, the exercised groups show improved immunity from infectious bacteria and fewer negative effects from stress.

A particularly good form of exercise is walking, since it relaxes and increases the overall circulation in the body and brain. Vigorous exercise will clear the stress hormones from your system and will send oxygen and glucose to the muscles that need it—thus limiting the amount available to the brain. Therefore, walking can actually increase your thought processes.

Get a Massage. A massage can calm both your mind and your muscles. Studies reveal that massages lower the levels of stress hormones in mothers with infants and also correct sleep patterns and reduce the negative effects of stress. Some people find relief with a simple, self-administered foot massage. Find a shallow box and fill it with one layer of golf balls. Have a seat, take your shoes off, and roll your feet over the golf balls.

Get Some Sleep

A proper amount of sleep is vital for optimal brain function. Stressful episodes can disrupt sleep cycles. People deprived of sleep usually show reduced mental performance. Long-term sleep loss can increase the severity of age-related diseases such as memory loss, obesity, diabetes, and high blood pressure. Some researchers have stated that "one complete night of sleep deprivation is as impairing in stimulated driving tests as a legally intoxicating blood level."

In general, overstressed people have difficulty sleeping and have disrupted sleep patterns. However, as men age, stress alone may lead to disrupted sleep. The emerging picture is that, as men become older, they react more sensitively to the stress hormone corticotropin-releasing hormone (CRH). CRH has stimulating effects and increases the alertness necessary to the body's responses to stress, but it's bad news for a good night's sleep. One study showed that when young and middle-aged men were given CRH, the older men consistently required more time to fall asleep and experienced less deep sleep. These findings suggest that increased incidence of sleep disorders in people of middle age likely resulted from an increased sensitivity to energizing stress hormones. Other studies have found that insomniacs released the highest levels of cortisol in the evening hours, compared with a group without sleep disorders. This study shows that the

The Normal Sleep Cycle

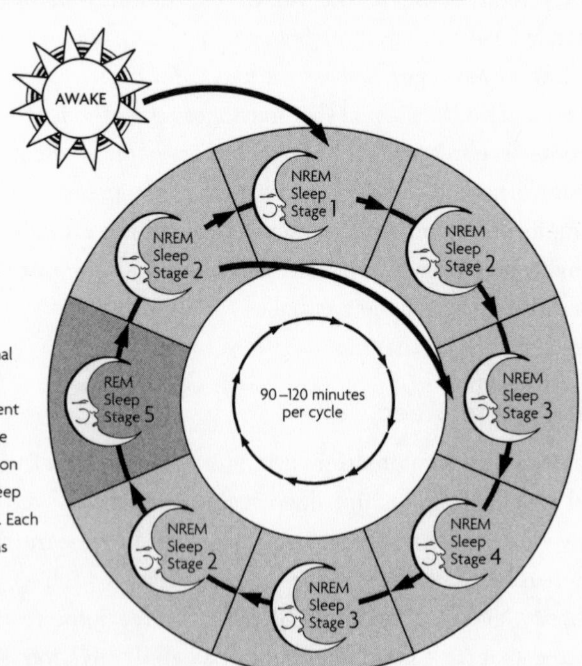

SLEEP STAGES
There are five stages in a normal sleep cycle. Stages 1 through 4 involve non-rapid eye movement (NREM). Stage 5 is the rapid eye movement (REM) stage. A person may complete five of these sleep cycles in a typical night's sleep. Each progressive cycle lasts longer as Stage 5 (REM stage) lengthens.

disorder insomnia actually results from uncontrolled stress hormones. Taking a quick twenty-minute nap might improve mental performance, especially after a sleepless night. Many studies show improved mental performances after a daytime nap.

Sleeping disorders are not all stress-related. An insidious condition called sleep apnea can rob one of sleep. Sleep apnea affects the breathing when muscles relax during sleep and the airflow is interrupted. This condition is often found in overweight people who have lost muscle tone from inactivity and/or aging. During sleep apnea, a person's airflow is temporarily blocked and, therefore, the blood's oxygen level plummets, which prompts the brain to cause the person to awaken enough to struggle and gasp for a breath. The person will often emit a loud snorting or snoring type of sound as he quickly inhales much-needed air into his lungs. People with sleep apnea can breathe normally in daily life but then experience this obstructive event hundreds of times over the course of one night's sleep. Thus, people with sleep apnea suffer from frequent awakening, loss of sleep cycles (see diagram), and poor mental functioning.

All animals sleep, yet why the brain requires sleep remains largely a mystery. However, researchers now believe sleep nurtures both brain development and the formation of memories. Studies show that an interrupted night of sleep affects learning and memory. Getting a good night's sleep, then, becomes crucial for preparing for a challenging presentation or examination. Both humans and animals perform poorly on memory tasks when sleep-deprived. Human sleep research shows that rapid eye movement (REM) sleep is critical for the formation of memories, and may prove necessary for learning how to perform certain mental tasks such as decision making or playing a musical instrument.

Step 6. Feed Your Brain with Physical Exercise

Relaxation and good health are essential prerequisites to creative thinking. We also need enough sleep to optimize our brainpower.

The body and mind should operate at peak efficiency with the benefits of a proper diet, rest, and exercise.

Heart-Smart Equals Brain-Gain

The health of your brain is directly tied to a proper amount of physical exercise. Walking particularly benefits your brain health since it elevates the general blood circulation rate and delivers more energy to the brain in the form of glucose and oxygen. Physical movement of the muscles from exercise increases the blood flow, which increases energy formation and the elimination of metabolic wastes. Exercise programs have been proven to stimulate the brain's blood vessels to grow, even in aged, previously sedentary animals.

Research has demonstrated that older citizens who walked on a regular basis displayed a significant increase in memory skills when compared with a group of physically inactive senior citizens. In addition, the risk of stroke was reduced by 57 percent in seniors who walked only twenty minutes per day. A number of studies have confirmed that older individuals who engage in regular physical exercise such as long walks have less age-related memory loss.

Researchers studied six thousand senior women over an eight-year period and discovered that the most active women in the group had much less cognitive decline. The women with the greatest activity level showed the most protection from memory decline, up to 40 percent compared with the inactive women. Moreover, the study showed the same results when other factors such as educational attainment, age, hormone replacement therapy use, and smoking status were taken into consideration.

In another study, physically inactive people between the ages of sixty and seventy years embarked on an exercise program. The study placed people into two groups. One group's exercises consisted of one-hour walks three times a week, while the other group performed stretching exercises and used light weights. The walkers showed a 5 to 7 percent increase in cardiovascular fitness that led to a 15 percent increased cognitive performance. The nonwalkers did not show any increase in mental functioning. Therefore, even in people aged seventy years and older, a regular walking program may benefit cognitive skills and improve memory.

Not only does physical activity seem to preserve cognitive functioning as people age, but it may even help forestall Alzheimer's disease. A study investigating five thousand men and women older than sixty-five found that those who regularly exercised were much more likely to retain their cognitive functions and developed less age-related dementia, including Alzheimer's. It appears that the more physically active a person is, the more they're protected from cognitive decline. Women in particular benefited more than men. Other studies have shown that women aged eighty-five and older have an 80 percent higher probability of having a better memory than men. Women at eighty-five years of age have much less cardiovascular disease than men of the same age. Actually, the sex differences in cardiovascular fitness may explain why older women tend to have better mental functioning than men. A healthy heart and vascular system maintain proper nutrient transport such as glucose to the brain and preserve mental function over a lifetime.

Benefits of Exercise on Brain Function

—Bathes the brain with nutrients in the form of glucose. The more glucose the brain uses, the more active it can be.

—Increases nerve connections to the brain.

—Increases oxygen in the bloodstream, which is then delivered to the brain.

—Releases endorphins into the bloodstream (creating the "runner's high").

—Relaxes the mind. The meditative rhythm of exercise allows your imagination and creativity to flow.

Exercise not only reduces the impacts of stressful situations, but it can also guard against depression and mood disorders. Researchers who tracked the moods of adults with an average age of seventy years found that those who consistently exercised had better moods ten years later than those participants who never exercised or stopped their exercise program. The physically inactive group had a greater incidence of depression and mood disorders. Another study in Finland also confirmed that exercise provides a vital, positive mental balance. People who decrease their levels of exercise in advanced age also risk having more symptoms of depression.

Exercise has also been shown to dramatically improve higher brain function such as planning and organization, as well as memory, attention, or concentration.

Appendix

Lifestyle Changes: Buy Better Brands

Whole Food Markets

These stores have a well-stocked inventory of whole, organic foods. Find the nearest location on their website: www.wholefoods.com.

Online or Mail-Order Organic Foods

Maranatha Natural Foods
P.O. Box 1046
Ashland, OR 97520
www.maranathanutbutters.com
Excellent organic nut butters

Walnut Acres Organic Farms
Penns Creek , PA 17862-0800
Phone: (800) 433-3998 (24 hours a day, 7 days a week)
www.walnutacres.com
Has many organic foods such as almond butter.

NAPA Organic Oils
Napa Valley Naturals c/o WorldPantry.com, Inc.
1024 Illinois Street
San Francisco, CA 94107
Phone: (866) 972-6879
Toll free: (415) 581-0067
Fax: (415) 581-0065
www.napavalleytrading.com

Spectrum Organic Products, Inc.
1304 South Point Blvd., Suite 280
Petaluma, CA 94954
Phone: (707) 778-8900
Toll free: (800) 995-2705
Fax: (707) 765-8470
Email: Info@SpectrumOrganic.com
www.spectrumnaturals.com
Organic expeller-pressed oils

Harvest Direct
P.O. Box 988
Knoxville, TN 37901-0988
Phone: (800) 835-2867

The Mail Order Catalog
P.O. Box 180
Summertown, TN 38483
Phone: (800) 695-2241

Dixie Diner's Club
7800 Amelia
Houston, TX 77055
Phone: (713) 688-4993

Eden Foods, Inc.
701 Tecumseh Road
Clinton, MI 49236

Natural Lifestyle
16 Lookout Drive
Asheville, NC 28804
Phone: (800) 752-2775

Green & Blacks Organic Chocolate
www.greenandblacks.com
Excellent organic 70 percent cocoa content dark chocolate

Organic Swiss Chocolate (Rapunzel)
Mercantile Food Company
P.O. Box SS
Philmont, NY 12565

Mail-Order Vitamins and Supplements

Pure Essence Laboratories, Inc.
P.O. Box 95397
Las Vegas, NV 89193
Phone: (888) 254-8000
Makes an excellent multivitamin.

NutriMedika Corp.
P.O. Box 733
Bayport, NY 11705
Phone: (800) 688-7462
Email: info@nutrimedika.com
Q-Gel®, a coenzyme Q10 supplement that has better absorption

Martek Biosciences Corporation
6480 Dobbin Road
Columbia, MD 21045
Phone: (410) 740-0081
Fax: (410) 740-2985
Email: info@martekbio.com
Neuromins (DHA)

Nutraceutical Corporation
1400 Kearns Blvd.
Park City, UT 84060
Phone: (800) 669-8877
Fax: (800) 767-8514
Email: products@nutraceutical.com
www.nutraceutical.com
Supplies the Solaray line of Leci-PS (phosphatidylserine) *and Neuromins (DHA)*

Solgar Vitamin and Herb
500 Willow Tree Road
Leonia, NJ 07605
Phone: (877) 765-4274
www.solgar.com
Supplies the Solgar line of Leci-PS (phosphatidylserine) and Neuromins (DHA)

Vitamin Research Products, Inc.
3579 Highway 50 East
Carson City, NV 89701
Phone: (800) 877-2447 (24 hours)
www.vrp.com
Lycopene supplements

Jason Natural Cosmetics
5500 W. 83rd Street
Los Angeles, CA 90045
Toll free (877) JASON-01, ext. 331
www.jason-natural.com
Email: jnp@jason-natural.com
Produces a line of excellent products. Try the Sea Fresh toothpaste!

Herbal Magic Roll-On Deodorant
Home Health Products for Life
Holbrook, NY 11741

Household Products, Cleaners

Seventh Generation, Inc.
212 Battery Street, Suite A
Burlington, VT 05401-5281
Phone: (802) 658-3773
Fax: (802) 658-1771
Toll-free (800) 456-1191
www.seventhgeneration.com
A company that specializes in nontoxic household cleaners. Their household cleaning products are specially formulated to be free of ammonia, chlorine, volatile organic chemicals, and other toxic chemicals.

Super Pine Cleaner
Available from www.realgoods.com
A natural pine oil cleaning agent that can be used to clean kitchens, counters, floors, and bathrooms

MIA Rose Products Inc.
Costa Mesa, CA 92626
Phone: (800) 292-6339
Citri-Glow, a citrus-based all-purpose cleaner

Fruit and Vegetable Wash

Organiclean TM
Walnut Acres (see Mail-Order Organic Foods)
Phone: (800) 433-3998

Water-Purifying Systems

Pūr Water Filters
Phone: (800) 787-5463
www.purwater.com
Manufacturers of water-filtering systems. Faucet-mounting, countertop, and under-sink varieties. Available through www.gaiam.com or www.realgoods.com.

The Health Store
P.O. Box 1727
West Palm Beach, FL 33402
www.thstore.com
Fax: (561) 686-5289
Email: CustomerService@thstore.com
Reverse osmosis is the most effective method of purifying water. Water is forced through semipermeable membranes, removing more than 98 percent of bacteria, viruses, chlorine, and toxic heavy metals. A Swedish company (www.electrolux.com) makes a high-quality, reverse osmosis system. The Electrolux RO 300 is a reverse osmosis purifier, compact enough to install under the kitchen sink. It does not have a tank; instead, when activated, it provides a direct and continuous flow of pure water. Available from The Health Store, above.

Air Filters

Real Goods
360 Interlocken Blvd., Suite 300
Broomfield, CO 80021-3440
Phone: (800) 762-7325
Fax: (800) 508-2342
www.realgoods.com
HEPA filters remove small invisible particulates from the air. BlueAir HEPA Air Filters are so effective in reducing airborne contaminates they are commonly used in European hospitals. Sun Pure Ultraviolet Air Purifier also removes viruses, bacteria, and toxic gases. It has a six-stage process that includes prefilters, carbon filters, HEPA filters, ionizers, and UV purifiers. Both are available from Real Goods.

Healthmate HEPA Air Filter
A highly rated portable HEPA filter. Available through www.gaiam.com.

Forced Air Vent Filters

Used as filters for air ducts. Available at www.gaiam.com.

Upright HEPA Vacuum Cleaner

A quiet unit that traps particulates down to 0.3 microns. Available at www.gaiam.com.

Personal Air Filter Face Masks

Greenscreen Air Filter Face Masks
3145 Geary Blvd., Suite 108
San Francisco, CA 94118
Phone: (415) 752-3200
Email: greenscreen@castleweb.com
Reduce exercise-induced asthma, prevent asthma, and avoid toxic dust, particulates, and environmental pollutant exposures with an air-filter face mask.

Lead Check Kits

HybriVet Systems, Inc.
P.O. Box 1210
Framingham, MA 01701
Phone: (800) 262-LEAD
Lead check swabs. Swabs will turn reddish pink if lead is present.

Water Testing Kits

WaterTest Corporation
New London, NH
Phone: (603) 526-6756
Water quality testing for lead.

PurTest™

This easy-to-use test kit is certified by an EPA laboratory and measures water for bacteria, lead, nitrates, nitrites, chlorine, copper, iron, pH, alkalinity, hardness, and hydro-

gen sulfide. Another kit tests for thirteen different pesticides. Available at www.gaiam.com or www.realgoods.com.

Trace Metal Analysis of Hair Samples

Biochemical Laboratories
P.O. Box 157
Edgewood, NM
Phone: (800) 545- 6562
While not an absolute measure of heavy metal exposure, trace metal analysis of hair can serve as a noninvasive means of qualitatively determining exposures to heavy metals.

Pesticide Alternatives

Tanglefoot™

Pet Guard™

TackTrap™

Drax™ Ant Baits

Bio-Neem™ Extract Taps

Real Goods
360 Interlocken Blvd. Suite 300
Broomfield, CO 80021-3440
Phone: (800) 762-7325
Fax: (800) 508-2342
www.realgoods.com

Orange Guard
Phone: (888) 659-3217
www.orangeguard.com
Controls insects on contact with natural extracts from orange peels (d-limonene) that disrupts the insect's respiratory system. Approved for use in organic gardens.

Bug Lightbulb

This fluorescent lightbulb does not attract most insects.

Solar Moler

A solar-powered unit that generates sonic waves to control moles safely.

Solar Anti Mosquito Guard

Repels mosquitoes with a high-frequency audible wave.

Dual Pest Control and Transonic Pest Control

Repel insects, mice, bats, fleas, spiders, ticks, moths with sonic waves. Available at www.gaiam.com.

Fruit Fly Trap

Uses a nontoxic insect attractant to trap fruit flies. Available at www.gaiam.com.

Pantry Moth Trap

Attracts and traps insects on a sticky surface. Available at www.gaiam.com.

Bug Off Instant Screen

A mesh screen that installs in minutes to protect against insects. Available at www.gaiam.com.

Weather Affects

3 Bud Way, Suite 29
Nashua, NH 03063
Phone: (800) 317-3666. Order 24 hours a day.
www.weatheraffects.com/5150.htm
Email: weatheraffects@aol.com.
Mosquito Trap. Uses the natural mosquito attractant CO_2 to trap mosquitoes.

Beneficial Insect Suppliers

Gardens Alive!
5100 Schenley Place
Lawrenceberg, IN
Phone: (812) 537-8650
Directory of suppliers of Beneficial Insects

Bio-Integral Resource Center
P.O. Box 7414
Berkeley, CA 94707
Phone: (510) 524-2567

Peaceful Valley Farm Supply
P.O. Box 2209
Grass Valley, CA 95945
Phone: (916) 272-4769

Ricon Vitova Beneficial Insectaries
P.O. Box 1555
Ventura, CA 93002
Phone: (805) 643-5407

Island Seed and Feed
29 S. Fairview
Goleta, CA 93117

Bibliography

Chapter 1. The Brain's Gatekeeper

Jacobson, J.L., and S.W. Jacobson. "Intellectual Impairment in Children Exposed to Polychlorinated Biphenyls in Utero." *New England Journal of Medicine* 335 (1996): 783–789.

Semchuk, K.M., E.J. Love, and R.G. Lee. "Parkinson's Disease and Exposure to Agricultural Work and Pesticide Chemicals." *Neurology* 42 (1992): 1328–1335.

Stephenson, J. "Exposure to Home Pesticides Linked to Parkinson Disease." *Journal of the American Medical Association* 283 (2000): 3055.

Chapter 2. Traffic Control: Letting in the Brain Boosters

Clauberg, M., and J.G. Joshi. "Regulation of Serine Protease Activity by Aluminum: Implications for Alzheimer Disease." *Proceedings of the National Academy of Sciences of the United States of America* 90 (1993): 1009–1012.

Detre, Z., et al. "Studies on Vascular Permeability in Hypertension: Action of Anthocyanosides." *Clinical Physiology and Biochemistry* 4 (1986): 143–149.

Havsteen, B. "Flavonoids, A Class of Natural Products of High Pharmacological Potency." *Biochemical Pharmacology* 32 (1983): 1141–1148. Commentary.

Kamal, A., A. Almenar-Queralt, et al. "Kinesin-Mediated Axonal Transport of a Membrane Compartment Containing β-Secretase and Presenilin-1 Requires APP." *Nature* 414 (2001): 643–648. Letters to *Nature*.

Maher, T.J., and R. Wurtman. "Possible Neurologic Effects of Aspartame, a Widely Used Food Additive." *Environmental Health Perspectives* 75 (1987): 53–57.

Robert, A.M., et al. "Action of Anthocyanosides of *Vaccinium myrtillis* on the Permeability of the Blood Brain Barrier." *Journal of Medicine* 8 (1977): 321–332.

Tixier, J.M., et al. "Evidence by In Vivo and In Vitro Studies That Binding of Pycnogenols to Elastin Affects Its Rate of Degradation by Elastases." *Biochemical Pharmacology* 33 (1984): 3933–3939.

Vazquez-Laslop, N., E.E. Zheleznova, et al. "Recognition of Multiple Drugs by a Single Protein: A Trivial Solution of an Old Paradox." *Biochemical Society Transactions* 28 (2000): 517–520.

Chapter 3. Red Light: Avoiding the Toxic Agents

Boyd, C.A. , M.H. Weiler, and W.P. Porter. "Behavioral and Neurochemical Changes Associated With Chronic Exposure to Low-Level Concentration of Pesticide Mixtures." *Journal of Toxicology and Environmental Health* 30 (1990): 209–221.

Chesters, G., and L.J. Schierow. "A Primer on Non-Point Pollution." *Journal of Soil and Water Conservation* 40 (1985): 14–18.

Creasey, W.A., and S.E. Malawista. "Monosodium L-Glutamate-Inhibition of Glucose Uptake in Brain as a Basis for Toxicity." *Biochemistry and Pharmacology* 20 (1971): 2917–2920.

Fleming, L., J.B. Mann, J. Bean, T. Briggle, and J.R. Sanchez-Ramos. "Parkinson's Disease and Brain Levels of Organochlorine Pesticides." *Annals of Neurology* 36 (1994): 100–103.

Hertzman, C., et al. "Parkinson's Disease: A Case-Control Study of Occupational and Environmental Risk Factors." *American Journal of Industrial Medicine* 17 (1990): 349–355.

Hong, S., J.P. Candelone, C.C. Patterson, and C.F. Boutron. "Greenland Ice Evidence Hemispheric Lead Pollution Two Millennia Ago by Greek and Roman Civilizations." *Science* 265 (1994): 1841–1843.

Jensen, A.A. "Transfer of Chemical Contaminants into Human Milk." In: Jensen, A.A., and S. A. Slorach, eds. *Chemical Contaminants in Human Milk*. Boca Raton, Fla: CRC Press, pp. 9–19, 1991.

Kass, D.A., E.P. Shapiro, et al. "Improved Arterial Compliance by a Novel Advanced Glycation End-Product Crosslink Breaker." *Circulation* 104 (2001): 1464.

Kittner, S.J., W.H. Giles, et al. "Homocyst(e)ine and Risk of Cerebral Infarction in a Biracial Population: The Stroke Prevention in Young Women Study." *Stroke* 30 (1999): 1554–1560.

Leong, C.W., N.I. Syed, and F.L. Lorscheider. "Retrograde Degeneration of Neurite Membrane Structural Integrity of Nerve Growth Cones Following In Vitro Exposure to Mercury." *NeuroReport* 12 (2001): 733–737.

Lovestone, S. "Is the Brain Another Site of End-Organ Damage?" *Neurology* 53 (1999): 1907.

Mason, R. "Understanding and Treating Toxic Overload: An Interview With Walter J. Crinnion, B.S., B.Th., N.D." *Alternative Complementary Therapies* 7 (2001):227–232.

Morris, M.S., P.F. Jacques, et al. "Hyperhomocysteinemia Associated With Poor Recall in the Third National Health and Nutrition Examination Survey." *American Journal of Clinical Nutrition* 73 (2001): 927–933.

Pimentel, D., and H. Lehman, eds. *The Pesticide Question: Environment, Economics, and Ethics*. New York: Chapman & Hall, 1993.

Pimentel, D., et al. "Environmental and Economic Cost of Pesticide Use." *BioScience* 42 (1992): 750–760.

Porter, W.P., et al. "Groundwater Pesticides: Interactive Effects of Low Concentrations of Carbamates Aldicarb and Methamyl and the Triazine Metribuzin on Thyroxine and Somatotropin Levels in White Rats." *Journal of Toxicology and Environmental Health* 40 (1993): 15–34

Rosman, K.J.R., W. Chisholm, S. Hong, C.F. Boutron, and J.P. Candelone. "Lead Isotope Record in Ancient Greenland Ice." 10th International Conference on Heavy Metals in the Environment, Hamburg, Germany, September 1995. 1 (1995): 34–36.

Schwartz, B.S., W.F. Stewart, K.I. Bolla, et al. "Past Adult Lead Exposure Is Associated With Longitudinal Decline in Cognitive Function." *Neurology* 55 (2000): 1144–1150.

Sechi, G.P. "Acute and Persistent Parkinsonism After Use of Diquat." *Neurology* 42 (1992): 261–263.

Semchuk, K.M., et al. "Parkinson's Disease and Exposure to Agricultural Work and Pesticide Chemicals." *Neurology* 42 (1992): 1328–1335.

Spence, J.D., V.J. Howard, L.E. Chambless, et al. "Vitamin Intervention for Stroke Prevention (VISP) Trial: Rationale and Design." *Neuroepidemiology* 20 (2001): 16–25.

U. S. Environmental Protection Agency. "Report to Congress: Nonpoint Source Pollution in the U. S. Office of Water Program Operations, Water Planning Division." Washington, D.C., 1984.

Chapter 4. Stress: The Unsuspected Environmental Toxic Agent

Arnsten, A.F., and P.S. Goldman-Rakic. "Noise Stress Impairs Prefrontal Cortical Cognitive Function in Monkeys: Evidence for a Hyper-dopaminergic Mechanism." *Archives of General Psychiatry* 55 (1998): 362–368

Biegler, R., A. McGregor, J.R. Krebs, and S.D. Healy. "A Larger Hippocampus Is Associated With Longer-Lasting Spatial Memory." *Proceedings of the National Academy of Sciences, United States of America* 98 (2001): 6941–6944.

Bosch, J.A., E.J.C. De Geus, A. Kelder, E.C.I. Veerman, J. Hoogstraten, and A.V.N Amerongen. "Differential Effects of Active Versus Passive Coping on Secretory Immunity." *Psychophysiology* 38 (2001): 836–846.

de Quervain, D.J.F., B. Roozendaal, R.M. Nitsch, J.L. McGaugh, and C.Hock. "Acute Cortisone Administration Impairs Retrieval of Long-Term Declarative Memory in Humans." *Nature Neuroscience* 3 (2000): 313–314.

Evans, G.W., and D. Johnson. "Stress and Open-Office Noise." *Journal of Applied Psychology* 85 (2000): 779–783.

Gould, E., A. Beylin, P. Tanapat, A. Reeves, and T.J. Shors. "Learning Enhances Adult Neurogenesis in the Hippocampal Formation." *Nature Neuroscience* 2 (1999): 260–265.

Petersen, R.C., C.R. Jack, Y.C. Xu, et al. "Memory and MRI-Based Hippocampal Volumes in Aging and AD." *Neurology* 54 (2000): 581–587.

Porter, N.M., and P.W. Landfield. "Stress Hormones and Brain Aging: Adding Injury To Insult?": *Nature Neuroscience* 1 (1998): 3–4.

Rhudy, J.L., and M.W. Meagher. "Noise Stress and Human Pain Thresholds: Divergent Effects in Men and Women." *Journal of Pain* 2 (2001): 57–64.

Roozendaal, B., R.G. Phillips, A.E. Power, S.M. Brooke, R.M. Sapolsky, and J.L. McGaugh. "Memory Retrieval Impairment Induced by Hippocampal CA3 Lesions Is Blocked by Adrenocortical Suppression." *Nature Neuroscience* 4 (2001): 1169–1171.

Taylor, S.E., L.C. Klein, B.P. Lewis, T.L. Gruenewald, R.A.R. Gurung, and J.A.Updegraff. "Biobehavioral Responses to Stress in Females: Tend-and-Befriend, Not Fight-or-Flight." *Psychological Review* 107 (2000): 411–429.

Xu, Y., C.R. Jack, P.C. O'Brien, et al. "Usefulness of MRI Measures of Entorhinal Cortex Versus Hippocampus in AD." *Neurology* 54 (2000): 1760–1767.

Chapter 5. A Feast for the Mind

Carlson, S.E., S.H. Werkman, P.G. Rhodes, and E.A. Tolley. "Visual-Acuity Development in Healthy Preterm Infants: Effect of Marine-Oil Supplementation." *American Journal of Clinical Nutrition* 58 (1993): 35–42.

Correa Leite, M.L., A. Nicolosi, et al. "Nutrition and Cognitive Deficit in the Elderly: A Population Study." *European Journal of Clinical Nutrition* 55 (2001): 1053–1058.

Eberhardt, M.V. , C.Y. Lee, and R.H. Liu. "Nutrition: Antioxidant Activity of Fresh Apples." *Nature* 405 (2000): 903–904.

Grandgirard, A., J.M. Bourre, R. Julliard, et al. "Incorporation of Trans Long-Chain N-3 Polyunsaturated Fatty Acids In Rat Brain Structure and Retina." *Lipids* 29 (1994): 251–258.

Joseph, J.A., B. Shukitt-Hale, et al. "Reversals of Age-Related Declines in Neuronal Signal Transduction, Cognitive, and Motor Behavioral Deficits with Blueberry, Spinach, or Strawberry Dietary Supplementation." *Journal of Neuroscience* 19 (1999): 8114–8121.

Kalmijn, S., E.J. Feskens, L.J. Launer, and D. Kromhout. "Polyunsaturated Fatty Acids, Antioxidants, and Cognitive Function in Very Old Men." *American Journal of Epidemiology* 145 (1997): 33–41.

Richards M., R. Hardy, et al. "Birth Weight and Cognitive Function in the British 1946 Birth Cohort: Longitudinal Population Based Study." *British Journal of Medicine* 322 (2001): 199–203.

Solfrizzi, V. , F. Panza, F. Torres, et al. "High Monounsaturated Fatty Acids Intake Protects Against Age-Related Cognitive Decline." *Neurology* 52 (1999): 1563.

Tang, M.X., D. Jacobs, et al. "Effect of Oestrogen During Menopause on Risk and Age at Onset of Alzheimer's Disease." *Lancet* 348 (1996): 429–431.

Willats, P., J.S. Forsyth, et al. "Effects of Long-Chain Polyunsaturated Fatty Acids in Infant Formula on Problem Solving at 10 Months of Age." *Lancet* 352 (1998) : 688–691.

Chapter 6. Eat to Beat the Blues

Bell, G.H., J.N. Davidson, and H. Scarborough. *Textbook of Physiology and Biochemistry*, 4th ed. London: Livingstone, 1954, p.167.

Benton, D., Brett, V., and Brain, P.F. "Glucose Improves Attention and Reaction to Frustration in Children." *Biological Psychology* 24 (1987): 95–100.

Bolton, R. "Aggression and Hypoglycemia among the Quolla: A Study in Psycho-biological Anthropology." *Ethology* 12 (1973): 227–257.

Bottiglieri, T., et al. "S-adenosylmethionine in Depression and Dementia: Effects of Treatment with Parenteral and Oral S-adenosylmethionine." *Journal of Neurology, Neurosurgery, and Psychiatry* 53 (1990): 1096–1098.

Bremner, J.D., M. Narayan, et al. "Hippocampal Volume Reduction in Major Depression." *American Journal of Psychiatry* 157 (2000): 115–118.

Deijen, J.B., M.L. Heemstra, and J.F. Orlebeke. "Dietary Effects on Mood and Performance." *Journal of Psychiatric Research* 23 (1989): 275–283.

Goldfarb, S. "Diet and Nephrolithiasis." *Annual Review of Medicine* 45 (1994): 235–241.

Gonder-Frederick, L.A., Cox, D.J., Bobbitt, S.A., and Pennebaker, J.W. "Mood Changes Associated with Blood Glucose Fluctuations in Insulin-Dependent Diabetes Mellitus." *Health Psychology* 8 (1989): 45–49.

Keith, R.E., O'Keefe, K.A., Blessing, D.L., and Wilson, D.G. "Alternations in Dietary Carbohydrate, Protein and Fat Intake and Mood State in Trained Female Cyclists." *Medicine and Science in Sports and Exercise* 23 (1991): 212–216.

Linkswiler, H.M., Zemel, M.B., Hegsted, M., and Schutte,S. "Protein-Induced Hypercalciuria." *Federal Proceedings* 40 (1981): 2429–2433.

Maesa, M., R. Smith, et al. "Fatty Acid Composition in Major Depression: Decreased ω3 Fractions in Cholesteryl Esters and Increased

C20: 4ω6/C20: 5ω3 Ratio in Cholesteryl Esters and Phospholipids." *Journal of Affective Disorders* 38 (1996): 35–46.

National Academy of Sciences. *Recommended Dietary Allowances*, 8th ed. Washington, D.C., 1974, p. 43.

Harding, M.G. Editorial. *The Lancet, Journal of the British Medical Association* 2 (1959): 956.

Osborn, T. "Amino Acids in Nutrition and Growth," *Journal of Biological Chemistry* 17 (1914): 325.

Owens, D.S., P.Y. Parker, and D. Benton. "Blood Glucose and Subjective Energy Following Cognitive Demand." *Physiology and Behavior* 62 (1997): 471–478.

Rosenthal, N.E., M.J. Genhart, B. Caballero, et al. "Psychobiological Effects of Carbohydrate- and Protein-Rich Meals in Patients With Seasonal Affective Disorder and Normal Controls." *Biological Psychiatry* 25 (1989): 1029–1040.

Scahill, L., P. B. Chappell, et al. "A Placebo-Controlled Study of Guanfacine in the Treatment of Children With Tic Disorders and Attention Deficit Hyperactivity Disorder." *American Journal of Psychiatry* 158 (2001): 1067–1074.

Scrimshaw, N. "An Analysis of Past and Present Recommended Daily Allowance for Protein in Health and Disease." *New England Journal of Medicine* 294 (1976): 200.

U.S.D.A. Agriculture Handbook, No.456.

Virkkunen, M. "Insulin Secretion During the Glucose Tolerance Test Among Habitually Violent and Impulsive Offenders." *Aggressive Behavior* 12 (1986): 303–310.

Virkkunen, M. "Insulin Secretion During the Glucose Tolerance Test in Antisocial Personality." *British Journal of Psychiatry* 142 (1983): 598–604.

Wurtman, J.J., A. Brzezinski, R.J. Wurtman, and B. Laferrere. "Effect of Nutrient Intake on Pre-menstrual Depression." *American Journal of Obstetrics and Gynecology* 161 (1989): 1228–1234.

Wurtman, R.J., F. Hefti, and E. Melamed, "Precursor Control of Neuromessenger Synthesis." *Pharmacological Reviews* 32 (1981): 315–335.

Chapter 7. Defending the Castle

Ahles, T.A., et al. "Neuropsychologic Impact of Standard-Dose Systemic Chemotherapy in Long-Term Survivors of Breast Cancer and Lymphoma." *Journal of Clinical Oncology* 20 (2002): 485–493.

Aschner, M. "Methyl Mercury Uptake across Bovine Brain Capillary Endothelial Cells in Vitro: The Role of Amino Acids." *Pharmacological Toxicology* 64 (1989): 293–297.

Aschner, M., and J.L. Aschner. "Mercury Neurotoxicity: Mechanisms of Blood-Brain Barrier Transport." *Neuroscience and Biobehavioral Reviews* 14 (1990): 169–176.

Couet, C., P. Jan, and G. Debry. "Lactose and Cataracts in Humans: A Review." *Journal of the American College of Nutrition* 10 (1991): 79–86.

Cramer, D.W., B.L. Harlow, W.C. Willett, et al. "Galactose Consumption and Metabolism in Relation to the Risk of Ovarian Cancer." *Lancet* 2 (1989): 66–71.

Cummings, J.L., and G. Cole. "Alzheimer Disease." *Journal of the American Medical Association* 287 (2002): 2335–2338.

Engelhart, M., et al. "Dietary Intake of Antioxidants and Risk of Alzheimer Disease." *Journal of the American Medical Association* 287 (2002): 3223–3229.

Gauthier, E., et al. "Environmental Pesticide Exposure as a Risk Factor for Alzheimer's Disease: A Case-Control Study." *Environmental Research,* Section A 86 (2001): 37–45.

Harris, W.R., G. Berthon, J.P. Day, et al. "Speciation of Aluminum in Biological Systems." *Journal of Toxicology and Environmental Health* 48 (1996): 543–568.

Jansson, E. "Aluminum Exposure and Alzheimer's Disease." *Journal of Alzheimer's Disease* 3 (2001): 541–549.

Kerper, L., et al. "Methylmercury Transport Across the Blood-Brain Barrier by an Amino Acid Carrier." *American Journal of Physiology* 5 (1992): 761–765.

Kruman, T., et al. "Folic Acid Deficiency and Homocysteine Impair DNA Repair in Hippocampal Neurons and Sensitize Them to Amyloid Toxicity in Experimental Models of Alzheimer's Disease." *Journal of Neuroscience* 22 (2002): 1752–1762.

Le Bars, P.L., et al. "A Placebo-Controlled, Double-Blind, Randomized Trial of an Extract of *Ginkgo biloba* for Dementia." *Journal of the American Medical Association* 278 (1997): 1327–1332.

Meyer, J.S., G.M. Rauch, R.A. Rauch, A. Haque, and K. Crawford. "Cardiovascular and Other Risk Factors for Alzheimer's Disease and Vascular Dementia." *Annals of the New York Academy of Sciences* 903 (2000): 411–423.

Mitchell, H.S., and W.M. Dodge. "Cataract in Rats Fed High-Lactose Rations." *Journal of Nutrition* 9 (1935): 37–49.

Rock, C., et al. "Increased Blood Mercury Levels in Patients with Alzheimer's Disease." *Journal of Neural Transmission* 105 (1998): 59–68.

Rondeau V., et al. "Relation between Aluminum Concentrations in Drinking Water and Alzheimer's Disease: An 8-Year Follow-Up Study." *American Journal of Epidemiology* 152 (2000): 59–66.

Sano M., et al. "A Controlled Trial of Selegiline, Alpha-Tocopherol, or Both as Treatment for Alzheimer's Disease." *New England Journal of Medicine* 336 (1997): 1216–1222.

Schweain, S.L. "Ginkgo." *Review of Natural Products* March 1998, p. 5.

Siegel N., and A. Hagu. "Aluminum Interaction with Calmodulin: Evidence for Altered Structure and Function from Optical Enzymatic Studies." *Biochimica et Biophysica Acta* 744 (1997): 36–45.

Simoons, F.J. "A Geographic Approach to Senile Cataracts: Possible Links with Milk Consumption, Lactase Activity and Galactose Metabolism." *Digestive Diseases and Sciences* 27 (1982): 257–264.

Skoog, I. "The Relationship between Blood Pressure and Dementia: A Review." *Biomedicine and Pharmacotherapy* 51 (1997): 367–375.

Sparks, D.L., et al. "Link between Heart Disease, Cholesterol, and Alzheimer's Disease: A Review." *Microscopy Research and Technique* 50 (2000): 287–290.

Varadarajan, S., S. Yatin, M. Aksenova, and D.A. Butterfield. "Review: Alzheimer's Amyloid Beta-Peptide-Associated Free Radical Oxidative Stress and Neurotoxicity." *Journal of Structural Biology* 130 (2000):184–208.

Part III: The 6-Step Brain-Purifying Program

Agency for Toxic Substances and Disease Registry. "Toxicological Profile for Trichloroethylene (TCE)." 1993.

Friedland, R.P., T. Fritsch, et al. "Patients with Alzheimer's Disease Have Reduced Activities in Midlife Compared with Healthy Control-Group Members." *Proceedings of the National Academy of Sciences of the United States of America* 98 (2001): 3440–3445.

Khatri, P., J.A. Blumenthal, et al. "Effects of Exercise Training on Cognitive Functioning Among Depressed Older Men and Women." *Journal of Aging and Physical Activity* 9 (2001): 43–57.

Krakow, B., M. Hollifield, et al. "Imagery Rehearsal Therapy for Chronic Nightmares in Sexual Assault Survivors With Posttraumatic Stress Disorder: A Randomized Controlled Trial." *Journal of the American Medical Association* 286 (2001): 537–545.

Maguire, E.A., et al. "Routes to Remembering: The Brains Behind Superior Memory." *Nature Neuroscience* 6 (2003): 90–95.

Mastropieri, M.A., and T.E. Scruggs. *Teaching Students Ways To Remember: Strategies for Learning Mnemonically.* Cambridge, Mass: Brookline Press, 1991.

Peltonen, R., J. Kjeldsen-Kragh, M. Haugen, et al. "Changes of Faecal Flora in Rheumatoid Arthritis During Fasting and One-Year Vegetarian Diet." *British Journal of Rheumatology* 33 (1994): 638–643.

Schneider, J.S., M.H. Leeb, D.W. Andersona, L. Zuckb, and T.I. Lidsky. "Enriched Environment During Development Is Protective Against Lead-Induced Neurotoxicity." *Brain Research* 896 (2001): 48–55.

Scruggs, T.E., and M.A. Mastropieri. "Classroom Applications of Mnemonic Instruction: Acquisition, Maintenance, and Generalization." *Exceptional Children* 58 (1992): 219–229.

Scruggs, T.E., and M.A. Mastropieri. "Reconstructive Elaborations: A Model for Content Area Learning." *American Educational Research Journal* 26 (1990): 311–327.

Spiegel, K., R. Leproult, and E. Van Cauter. "Impact of Sleep Debt on Metabolic and Endocrine Function." *Lancet* 354 (1999): 1435–1439.

Verhaeghen, P., and A. Marcoen. "On the Mechanisms of Plasticity in Young and Older Adults After Instruction in the Method of Loci: Evidence for an Amplification Model." *Psychology of Aging* 11 (1996): 164–178.

Williams, K.A., M.M. Kolar, et al. "Evaluation of a Wellness-based Mindfulness Stress Reduction Intervention: A Controlled Trial." *American Journal of Health Promotion* July/August 2001.

Yaffe, K., D. Barnes, et al. "A Prospective Study of Physical Activity and Cognitive Decline in Elderly Women: Women Who Walk." *Archives of Internal Medicine* 161 (2001): 1703–1708.

Index

E

F

N

Q

R

S

W

Z